Fibromyalgia

A Handbook for
Self Care & Treatment

Janet A. Hulme, M.A., P.T.

Foreword by
Peggy Schlesinger, M.D.
Rheumatologist

Fibromyalgia, A Handbook for Self Care & Treatment

ISBN Number: 1-928812-01-5

Design & Layout
Gateway Printing
Missoula, Montana

Published in the U.S.A. by
Phoenix Publishing Co.
P.O. Box 8231
Missoula, Montana 59807

Acknowledgements

There are many individuals to thank for this new edition. My heartfelt thanks to Catherine Goodman, P.T., Candace and Cecily Ryan, Jane Emery, Kathleen Miller, Susie Risho, Debra Sommer, Kim Ericsson, and Eloyce Kockler for reading and offering their expert suggestions as the book took shape. I am always grateful to Donna Elliott for typing and formatting this manuscript. I am forever thankful to my family Erika, Abigail, and Richard Hulme, and John Bower who edit, offer cirtical guidance, and tolerate my isolation as I write. Finally, I am indebted to all my patients for providing essential information about what works and more importantly what does not.

The information and procedures contained in this book are based upon the research and the personal and professional experiences of the author. They are not intended as a substitute for consulting with your physician or other health care provider. The publisher and author are not responsible for any adverse effects or consequences resulting from the use of any of the suggestions, preparations, or procedures discussed in this book. All matters pertaining to your physical health should be supervised by a health care professional.

Other publications
by the author

Managing Fibromyalgia
A Six Week Course in Self Care
Author: Barbara Penner, M.S., P.T.
Contributions by Janet A. Hulme, M.A., P.T.

Beyond Kegels
Fabulous four exercises and more...
to prevent and treat incontinence

Beyond Kegels Book II
Treatment Algorithms
&
Special Populations

Geriatric Incontinence
A Behavioral and Exercise Approach
to Treatment

Table of Contents

Foreword

Fibromyalgia is a chronic painful condition of epidemic propor-
tions. The associated disability that fibromyalgia patients experience
often takes a significant toll on their emotional and family life, their
vocational choices, and their finances. The techniques of self care
explained in detail in this book offers individuals with fibromyalgia a
way to focus their energies in a positive way, working to improve
symptoms and reduce their disease related disability. In this book, Jan
presents a well written understandable approach to monitoring
symptoms and responding with appropriate therapeutic intervention.
Although her techniques and theories may not be as firmly rooted in a
traditional medical model, the results speak for themselves. She believes
firmly, as do I, that learning about one's illness and learning how to
care for oneself are vitally important steps to achieve control over this
chronic disease before it controls you. I hope you find help in this
book to get started on the path of healing.

Peggy Schlesinger, M.D.
Rheumatologist

PART 1: WHAT IS IT? DO I HAVE IT?

Chapter 1
Introduction

The Mystery

Janet A. Hulme, P.T.

Fibromyalgia (FMS) has been termed the mystery condition in that the symptoms are not measurable by the usual medical tests like X-rays and blood tests. The symptoms are multiple instead of one or two defined entities. The severity may vary within one individual depending on the time of day and time of year. For these and other reasons physicians and their patients question the diagnosis. For example, Jody, a computer programmer, tells her husband she doesn't believe the physician's diagnosis of fibromyalgia is correct for the headaches, shoulder, neck and arm pain she is experiencing. Dr. Malone comments to colleagues that fibromyalgia is a garbage can diagnosis used when no other diagnosis fits the individual's symptoms. Dr. Sage tells patients there is no such thing as fibromyalgia, that the symptoms are caused by biochemical abnormalities in the brain and should be treated with antidepressant medications. All these individuals are caring, competent and conscientious, but confused about the diagnosis. It is a mystery.

Confusing Signs and Symptoms

Any individual with fibromyalgia can be very confused and frustrated by the symptoms as well as the information he/she may receive from the medical profession. "Is it important to take the pain and fatigue seriously? Or should I ignore it and get on with my life the best I can?" are questions often asked. The widespread chronic muscle pain can mimic the pain of disc problems, sciatica, tendinitis, bursitis or nerve compression. It can mimic the pain of cancer or a heart problem even though all tests for those conditions return normal. The physician and individual are left with the reality of pain that significantly changes life patterns but not medical tests to confirm what it is or what to do.

The usual blood tests, X-rays, and other medical tests are negative in FMS. While these tests indicate that other diagnoses are not causing the pain and associated symptoms the individual describes, when they are taken as the final word that there is nothing wrong, the conclusion is that this individual's symptoms are "all in his/her head." The response to "mental" misperception is to ignore it, pretend it isn't there, or to use drugs to alter the mental perception. Even seemingly objective signs and symptoms of FMS can be confusing. The most common sign is tender points throughout the body. Some medical professionals will argue that the tender points are over acupressure points that are always tender in any individual. Others will state that the tender points are no different than trigger points in myofascial pain syndrome. The mystery often remains unsolved.

Associated Symptoms

Associated symptoms of fibromyalgia can be as important in the diagnosis as the pain and tender points. Yet they too can cause confusion. The associated symptoms include problems in the sensory systems of touch, hearing, sight, smell and taste; the muscle systems of arms, legs, and trunk; the heart, lungs, and circulatory systems; the stomach and intestinal systems and the brain and nervous system. The question is often asked, "How can one diagnosis cause all these very different problems?"

Mysterious too is the fact that these symptoms come and go in intensity. They can be more intense at times, limiting daily activities significantly. At other times the symptoms may be hardly noticeable.

What Is Normal?

Individuals with fibromyalgia describe growing up seeing family members with these symptoms and/or experiencing their own symptoms during childhood. They considered these symptoms as a "normal" part of being alive. Mary remembers abdominal discomfort and sleep disturbance since being a young child. "Everyone has gut pain, I just don't cope with it as well as others," she told her physician. Jane assumed that, "No one sleeps through the night and feels rested. I just don't deal with being tired as well as others." Ken commented to his physician, "All the men in my family have headaches, bad backs, and indigestion. That's normal." Since fibromyalgia often runs in families, individuals see parents and other relatives living with the symptoms and fail to diagnose their associated symptoms as FMS. "Normal" must be seen in a wider context, comparing the individual to a diverse and large population, not just their family group.

One Part of the Elephant or the Whole Thing

The difficulty in diagnosing and treating FMS comes when the individual or clinician looks at a local symptom rather than looking at the involvement of the entire body. Jody tells her doctor, "My low back and leg are so painful I can't walk, sit, or sleep." When her doctor asks for any other symptoms Jody neglects to mention there are any other problems because she doesn't relate her indigestion, headaches or cold hands to the back pain – those are just normal symptoms she and others in her family have all the time. "Just fix this back so I can get back to work," Jody begs her doctor. The physician seeing Jody does the usual X-rays and blood tests which come back normal. She concludes that this is a local muscle pull or strain and treats it with appropriate treatment for a musculoskeletal problem. Both Jody and her physician are frustrated when she doesn't improve or improves for a few days but then gets worse again.

The approach of looking only at the trunk of the elephant instead of at the whole elephant has historically been a problem in diagnosing and treating fibromyalgia. When the "whole elephant" is acknowledged the concept that this isn't a local problem leads to the treatment of the whole. Instead of treating a muscle or limb the treatment is directed towards the whole body. Fibromyalgia is like diabetes in this way. Diabetes affects every cell of the body. It affects eye function, brain function, muscle function, etc. Yet diabetes is not a "mental condition" occurring from a brain defect. Rather it is a problem primarily in the pancreas which then affects every other cell and function in the body. Fibromyalgia is more like diabetes than it is like tendinitis or myofascial pain syndrome.

Every Little Cell

Fibromyalgia affects every cell of the body. When the muscle, ligament, or tendon cells are significantly affected the symptoms are felt most in the arms, legs and back. Common medical diagnoses are tendinitis, bursitis, rotator cuff injury, ulnar nerve compression, carpal tunnel syndrome, back strain, or thoracic outlet syndrome. When the cells of the stomach, intestine, or uterus are affected the symptoms are felt in the abdomen and pelvis. Common medical diagnoses are premenstrual syndrome (PMS), interstitial cystitis, urethral syndrome, and irritable bowel syndrome. When the brain cells are significantly affected the symptoms are experienced in the thought, memory and mental/emotional areas. Common medical diagnoses include anxiety disorder, panic disorder, and depression. The important aspect to remember is that these symptoms are part of a widespread problem. The criteria for a local diagnosis may be met but the symptoms are part of a systemic problem that is resulting in the local symptoms. Treat the leg, arm or back and it may feel better for a short period of time but it isn't a permanent solution. Treat the underlying dysfunction and the arm, leg or back improves over the long term and the less dominant symptoms also improve over the long term.

The Cause

The question becomes "What is creating these multiple and varied fibromyalgia symptoms?" In diabetes it is known that the pancreas is dysfunctional and unable to produce insulin, a chemical essential to combine with sugars to provide the nutrients for energy production in all body cells. What is the comparable dysfunction in fibromyalgia? In this new century we are beginning to understand more about the underlying dysfunctions involved in fibromyalgia. Chapter 3 describes what is known and unknown about the cause and underlying dysfunction of fibromyalgia.

The Path to Best Results

Monitoring Internal Health

Like diabetes, at the present time we do not have a cure for fibromyalgia. Instead there is a need to carry out daily procedures that maintain the health of all cells of the body. So for diabetics it is necessary to take multiple blood glucose readings daily and then inject insulin or take pills multiple times a day. A special diet and exercise program is also needed. When these tests and self care techniques are used regularly individuals with diabetes can function in daily life side by side with their nondiabetic counterparts. It is possible to be whatever one wants to be: an Olympic athlete, an accountant, a logger, a parent, a teacher. The same often holds true for the individual with fibromyalgia.

Individuals with fibromyalgia must carry out daily tests and self care routines to maintain the health of all cells of the body. It is necessary to monitor signs and symptoms multiple times a day – for some it will be palpation of tender points, for others it will be blood glucose levels, others will need to monitor blood pressure and heart rate and for others it will be to monitor hand temperature. These tests indicate how the specific body systems are functioning. A summary of the tests, signs and symptoms helps the individual determine which fibromyalgia subcategories are appropriate. The summary of the tests, signs, and symptoms also directs the level and type of self care needed to maintain healthy functioning in daily life. It is again like diabetes, the monitoring tests tell the present status but cannot predict future status so regular monitoring is necessary. How often monitoring is required depends how volatile the condition is in both diabetes and fibromyalgia. Sometimes monitoring is required 4-5 times daily. Other individuals are able to maintain health monitoring 1-2 times daily. Neither diabetes nor fibromyalgia take the weekends or vacations off. It is a 7 day a week, 365 days a year maintenance effort. Chapter 11 describes the self monitoring system and how to decide which monitoring tests are important for you.

Subcategories – What Are They?

The issue remains "What can we do to alleviate the symptoms?" since, at the present time, we cannot cure this condition. The approach taken in this book is management through self care based on the general diagnosis of FMS and additionally on the subcategory each individual finds appropriate. For our purposes there are five subcategories of fibromyalgia on which to base self care, **Type 1, Type 2, Type 3, Type 4, and Type 5** (see Figure 1). These subcategories can be determined by using medical tests and relatively simple nonprescriptive test procedures (Chapter 11). Each type can be treated medically and with nonprescriptive methods in many cases. These are described in Chapters 12-25. The self care interventions are based on the subcategory symptoms and test results. The interventions are designed to maintain or rebalance body systems of the FMS individual on a daily basis.

FMS Subcategory Types

1   **Type 1**   Hypoglycemic Tendencies

2   **Type 2**   Hypothyroid Tendencies

3   **Type 3**   Neurally Mediated Hypotension Tendencies

4   **Type 4**   Immune System Dysfunction Tendencies

5   **Type 5**   Reproductive Hormone Dysfunction Tendencies

G   **Type G**   General Fibromyalgia Symptoms

Figure 1

The Solution

Self Care Stabilizing Loops

The usual approach to fibromyalgia management has been using medical intervention, medication and self care to address general symptoms of pain, fatigue, and sleep disturbance. The purpose of this book is to integrate the concept of subcategories and their self care stabilizing loops within fibromyalgia. This book describes how testing and treating within these subcategories can provide improved outcomes when combined with the more traditional treatment. The self care stabilizing loops are continuous cycles of assessment, treatment, measurement, and reassessment. When the subcategory dysfunctions specific to the individual are monitored on a continual basis and treated to maintain better homeostasis the FMS individual is able to accomplish work, exercise, and social functions with significantly decreased pain, fatigue and sleep disturbance. The FMS individual experiences increased endurance in exercise, work, and recreational endeavors where previously a glass ceiling seemed to prevent further progress in function. The subcategories are not new diagnoses, rather they are groupings of symptom tendencies. As tendencies rather than diagnoses each tendency can be affected through nonprescriptive strategies with resulting changes in symptoms. The initial intervention for FMS individuals should be with treatment for the general symptoms as described in Chapter 12. When these have been utilized to their maximum effectiveness, specific subcategory intervention can offer additional function and endurance. These strategies are described in Chapters 13-19. Some FMS individuals may have strong characteristics of more than one subcategory so that combining interventions becomes necessary. In all interventions the FMS individual is responsible for the monitoring as well as the daily life style changes. It is a life style change rather than a one time intervention with a cure, that restores function and quality of life to individuals with FMS.

Deserving the Royal Treatment

As Harry observes about Sally when she asks for her sandwich "with lettuce, no tomato, just a swish of mayonnaise and no mustard," "You are indeed high maintenance." Individuals with fibromyalgia symptoms are indeed high maintenance and deserving of it. A high maintenance individual deserves to have what he/she needs to keep well and healthy. The crux of the matter is often the word "deserve." It is more common for individuals in our culture to deny the needs of the body in deference to the mind's commands. The mind commands. "Do this, do that, faster, better." The mind often tells the body to "shut up and do what I tell you." The individual with fibromyalgia symptoms must turn that concept upside down. "What do you need body? I will listen and do what you need." If that is considered high maintenance in our culture so be it. It is the same need of the diabetic to monitor and respond to the body's needs to be able to function as a healthy unit of mind and body.

Fibromyalgia has been referred to as the Royalty Syndrome. The story is told that the royal families of Europe were used to a high maintenance life style. It was an expected norm that servants and musicians would provide for the individual desires of each prince or princess. Just look to the story of the Princess and the Pea. The princess could feel a pea under seven mattresses and kept adding mattresses until she could no longer feel the pea and could sleep through the night. She deserved it because she was a princess. It extended to servants fixing meals, providing clothing, massage, music, etc. that appealed to each individual royal prince, princess, king and queen. It was the expected norm of daily life. When Europeans moved to America, so the story goes, the Puritan ethic took over with the dogma of work, work, work, work, and deprivation as the way to exist and be pleasing to the Almighty. High maintenance was considered sinful and an impossible life style in this challenging new country. The prince or princess suffered in silence as the culture denied there was a prince or princess in any of us. Much of our culture and the medical establishment of managed care continues to deny this reality today.

High Maintenance

Solving the mystery of fibromyalgia means that individuals with symptoms are by definition "high maintenance" and deserve to develop the techniques of high maintenance that allow them to be relatively symptom free. High maintenance is defined as prioritizing the healthy state of body and mind such that taking the time for self assessment and care on a daily, sometimes even hourly basis, is the top priority. The highest priority for high maintenance individuals is to perform the necessary tasks that result in experiencing the healthiest state possible. Why? Because that will allow them to think clearly, take care of their daily functions independently, work in the home or work environment efficiently and effectively, have families, and interact socially and recreationally in a healthy long term way. Without the "high mainte-nance" individuals with fibromyalgia symptoms may be dependent and miserable. Society, family and friends will view them as sick. Sick or high maintenance – these are the choices. Each individual must decide for him/herself. This book is written for those who decide they want to be well and are willing to view themselves as high maintenance. They believe they deserve health and wellness and the time and effort it takes.

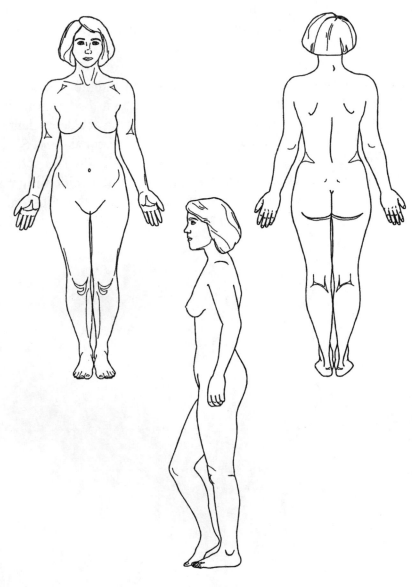

My Pain Pattern

Date_____

Chapter 2

What Are
The Symptoms?

Janet A. Hulme, P.T.

What Is It?

Fibromyalgia is defined as pain as opposed to inflammation of the soft tissues of the body. Soft tissues include muscles, tendons, ligaments and fascia.

Fibromyalgia is considered a syndrome and not a disease. It is a complex of symptoms rather than a pathological process that progresses over time. It is chronic in nature, the symptoms are present for more than three months duration before the diagnosis is made. Chronic, pervasive pain is the major complaint and is described by some as a migraine headache of the muscles. The diffuse pain is located on both sides of the body, with pain above and below the waist, in muscles of the face and neck, back and abdomen, arms and legs, hands and feet. FMS individuals also complain of fatigue and nonrestorative or nonrestful sleep. Draw in the pain you have experienced in the past two weeks on the diagram on page 10.

Myofascial Pain Syndrome and FMS

FMS is confused with myofascial pain syndrome at times. They are different entities. Fibromyalgia is systemic in nature while myofascial pain syndrome is a more localized phenomena. Fibromyalgia has characteristic tender points, localized areas that are painful when pressure is applied. Myofascial pain syndrome has characteristic trigger points that are locally painful but also refer pain to other areas when pressure is applied.

Physiological Components

Physiological components of the pain, stiffness, and fatigue of FMS can be demonstrated with the use of surface electromyography and thermography. Blood circulation to muscles of the back, arms, legs, hands and feet can be significantly decreased at rest. In some FMS individuals there is noticeable circulation decrease with barometric pressure changes. During exercise, circulation to muscles and the brain should normally increase, but in FMS just the opposite occurs. Transport of oxygen and food products to muscle cells and removal of waste products is compromised.

The resting level of muscle activity during standing and sitting, even reclining, is like the idle on a car engine and can be high or low. In an individual with FMS the muscles' resting level is generally high, the engine is on high idle all the time, which means that even at rest the muscles need more oxygen and food products and accumulate more waste products than normal.

During daily activities such as cleaning, cooking, typing, and even socializing the muscles used for these activities "overdo" or are at a higher level of activity than muscles of an individual without FMS doing the same tasks. Instead of floating through the activity or social situation the FMS individual's muscles tend to act like "a bull in a china closet" moving fast, strong, and not always in the right direction. The result is that the work gets done quickly, but the fallout is fatigue and pain on the part of the FMS individual.

When Rest Is Not Rest

Once the activity is over and the FMS individual is attempting to "rest," these same muscles continue to repeat the activity over and over again even though nothing outwardly is moving, i.e., the muscle activity is in the same pattern as during the activity but at a somewhat decreased level while the individual thinks he/she is resting "quietly." For example, the forearm muscles of any individual writing for several minutes will be highly active in a particular pattern. At completion of writing (hands resting in lap) a non-FMS forearm muscle group activity pattern would be quiet with little activity. The FMS muscle pattern with hands in lap would mimic the writing pattern but at a somewhat decreased amplitude even though the arms appeared to be still.

No wonder there is pain and aching for one to two days after a seemingly simple light activity. Those muscles kept doing the activity long after the conscious mind was on to another task.

A Small Stress – A Big Response

The activity of the FMS individual's heart, stomach, intestines, blood vessels and sweat glands during daily stressors tend to be excessive. The heart beats faster, the stomach contracts erratically, the smooth muscle of the intestines and bowel contracts abnormally, the breathing rate becomes erratic and rapid, and blood vessels constrict, decreasing blood flow to body parts at times. All these changes occur in response to a relatively mild life stressor. The FMS individual feels heart palpitations, shortness of breath, chest pains, coldness, sweating, numbness, tingling, even panic and anxiety that continues long after the event is over. These responses may linger even after cognitive memory of the initiating event is gone. Cellular memory, a previously suspected but now documented phenomena, may explain this.

When non-FMS individuals experience these changes the body responses occur in smaller amplitude and for a shorter period of time than the FMS individual. The non-FMS responses might include rapid breathing, feeling hot or cold, and feeling the heart beating for a few minutes to half an hour, but this is quickly followed by a return to normal. The FMS nervous system's subtleness of response is fragile with both the responses being more exaggerated and the return to a normal state taking more time.

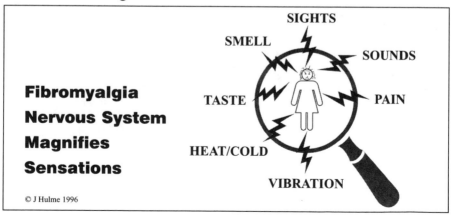

Fibromyalgia Nervous System Magnifies Sensations

SIGHTS
SMELL
SOUNDS
TASTE
PAIN
HEAT/COLD
VIBRATION

© J Hulme 1996

Figure 2

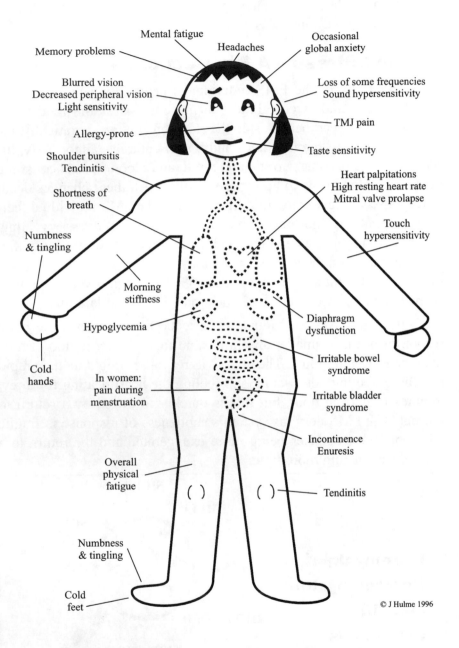

Mental fatigue

Memory problems

Headaches

Occasional global anxiety

Blurred vision
Decreased peripheral vision
Light sensitivity

Loss of some frequencies
Sound hypersensitivity

TMJ pain

Allergy-prone

Taste sensitivity

Shoulder bursitis
Tendinitis

Heart palpitations
High resting heart rate
Mitral valve prolapse

Shortness of
breath

Touch
hypersensitivity

Numbness
& tingling

Morning
stiffness

Diaphragm
dysfunction

Hypoglycemia

Irritable bowel
syndrome

Cold
hands

In women:
pain during
menstruation

Irritable bladder
syndrome

Incontinence
Enuresis

Overall
physical
fatigue

( )   ( )

Tendinitis

Numbness
& tingling

Cold
feet

© J Hulme 1996

Figure 3: Associated Symptoms of Fibromyalgia

Associated Symptoms

FMS is sometimes described as the "irritable everything" syndrome. Instead of quieting or inhibiting sensations, the FMS individual's nervous system magnifies sensory input. Sounds, light, touch, pressure, smell, taste, heat/cold, and pain can all be exaggerated by the FMS nervous system (Figure 2). Symptoms can be evident throughout the body, but some individuals will feel them in one area more than another (Figure 3).

Some periods of time there will be more symptoms, other times very few. Associated symptoms and the frequency with which they occur in FMS include:

Mental and physical fatigue 85%

This is overwhelming tiredness resulting in great effort or even inability to move through physical tasks. It can occur with or without precipitating events. Individuals describe mental fatigue, confusion, inability to problem solve or remember even simple sequences.

Sleep disturbance / morning fatigue 80%

Deep sleep or delta sleep is when body cells repair and replace themselves and essential hormones for growth and metabolism are released. Growth hormone in an FMS individual is produced in the greatest quantities in the early morning compared to a non-FMS individual who produces it throughout the night, so an FMS individual describes getting his/her best sleep in the morning when others are getting up. Eighty percent of growth hormone is released during deep sleep and growth hormone is essential for normal muscle metabolism and tissue repair. FMS individuals have significantly disrupted deep or Stage 4 sleep. It may take 1-2 hours to get to sleep. Any noise, smell, or other sensory stimuli may lead to arousal. Deep sleep can be disrupted by alpha wave sleep, awake-like brain waves, that intrude into deep sleep, so it is called alpha-delta sleep anomaly. For others sleep can be disrupted by restless leg syndrome or sleep apnea. The FMS individual sleeps restlessly, waking 2-29 times during the night and wakes feeling stiff, sore, and tired. Muscles maintain a high level of activity at rest, breathing continues to be shallow and erratic, and the circulatory system is often unstable which results in significantly decreasing body temperature as the night progresses. Hypoglycemia (low blood sugar) may cause night time arousal in FMS individuals.

By contrast, a non-FMS individual usually gets into bed, falls asleep in 15-30 minutes, and sleeps through the night. During deep sleep, muscles go into a relaxed state, breathing slows, and circulation maintains a stable body temperature. The individual wakes feeling rested, warm, and relaxed. Feeling tired and sore is not normal!

Morning stiffness 75%

This is the persistence of stiffness in the morning for more than 30 minutes. Stiffness can be the feeling of muscles, fascia, or even joints being glued down or jelling when the body is in one position for any period of time.

Global anxiety 72%

Individuals describe a feeling of anxiousness, irritability and over-concern without specific precipitating events. The individual describes a long list of problems – past, present, and potential.

Irritable bowel syndrome (IBS) 70%

Specific bowel complaints include alternating diarrhea and constipation, abdominal pain, abdominal gas, and nausea. Gut contractions are normally at six cycles/minute. However, in IBS they are at three cycles/minute which may give rise to the constipation and abdominal pain, followed by diarrhea. The enteric nervous system, which is the nervous system of the intestines, is involved in IBS.

Irritable bladder syndrome, female urethral syndrome 40%

Specific complaints include urgency, urinary frequency (as often as every 15-30 minutes), lower abdominal pain and pressure, incontinence (loss of urine), enuresis (night time loss of urine), and interstitial cystitis symptoms (pain and frequency of urination).

Headaches 70%

Migraine and tension-type headaches are frequent in FMS individuals. Migraine headaches produce one-sided, throbbing head pain often with associated nausea and hypersensitivity to light and sound. Tension headaches produce a sensation of tightness or pressure across the forehead, on both sides of the head, at the back of the neck, extending into the shoulders. Tension headaches are not necessarily caused by psychological stress or muscle tension.

Raynaud's phenomena 38%

Individuals describe cold hands and feet, color changes in tips of fingers and toes.

Sicca syndrome 33%

Individuals describe dry eyes and/or mouth.

Depression 20-50%

FMS is not a psychiatric disorder. Depression can occur in response to pain. Clinical depression is no more prevalent in FMS individuals than in the general population.

Paresthesias 50%

Individuals describe numbness and tingling in arms, legs, hands, and feet.

Subjective swelling 50%

Individuals describe subjective feeling of swelling, often in hands and feet. It is usually not observable by another person.

Pelvic pain 43%

Recurrent pain in the pelvic area related to FMS is often misdiagnosed as endometriosis and interstitial cystitis. Dysmenorrhea or painful menstruation is frequent with FMS. Pelvic and lower abdominal pain may be caused by dysfunction of the enteric nervous system or pelvic congestion (varicose veins in the pelvis). If an individual experiences varicose veins in the legs and/or has low blood pressure there may be a greater predisposition to pelvic congestion leading to pelvic/abdominal pain.

Temporomandibular dysfunction (TMD) 25%

TMD causes face and head pain. In FMS most of the problems are related to muscles and ligaments surrounding the jaw joint, not necessarily the joint itself.

Visual problems up to 95%

Individuals describe blurring, double vision, bouncing images.

Auditory problems 31%

At times certain frequencies are difficult for an individual with FMS to hear while at other times hypersensitivity to some frequencies is present.

Respiratory dysfunction 33%

Dyspnea or shortness of breath at rest and during physical activity is common. Irregular, erratic breathing patterns are predominant during maximal exertion.

Cognitive (memory) problems 71%

Decreased attention span, decreased concentration, and impaired short term memory can have significant implications for learning new behavior and remembering past learning. There may be more time needed to process information and/or increased repetitions to retain a skill.

Hypersensitivity to noise, odors, heat or cold 50-60%

There is magnification of environmental stimuli in the FMS individual. Incoming sensations are amplified, sensations from the skin, ears, eyes, nose, and/or mouth are perceived by the individual as excessive (Figure 2).

Clumsiness

Dropping objects, tripping, and running into things are common in FMS.

Mitral valve prolapse 75%

One of the heart valves bulges more than usual during the heart-beat. It may be that in most cases the prolapse is caused by an imbalance between the sympathetic and parasympathetic nerve impulses to the heart.

Restless Leg Syndrome (RLS); Periodic Leg Movement Disorder (PLMD) 30-60%

Symptoms described include rhythmic, uncontrolled leg movements, calf muscle cramping, feeling that legs are alive and unable to be still. Numbness, tingling and burning sensations may be present.

Allergies

There can be a history suggestive of hypersensitivity to environmental allergen.

Hypoglycemic tendencies 45-50%

Individuals describe weakness, tremors, irritability, anxiety, and mental disorientation. This may be particularly prevalent after exercise or during the night while sleeping.

Joint hypermobility 43%

Increased flexibility or looseness of joints, for example the thumb can touch the forearm and the elbow hyperextends.

Low Blood Pressure and High Resting Heart Rate. Neurally Mediated Hypotension (NMH) or Vasopressor Syncope 40%

Dizzy, light headedness, low blood pressure, and high resting heart rate are typical symptoms. The abnormal heart rate and blood pressure are caused by dysfunctional communication signals from the nervous and hormonal systems. The autonomic nervous system does not adequately respond to changes in heart rate and blood vessel constriction to maintain normal blood pressure.

On the following page is the General Fibromyalgia Criteria and Associated Symptoms Questionnaire. Check the appropriate boxes that describe your symptoms in the last two weeks.

General Fibromyalgia Criteria Questionnaire

Check off the appropriate boxes that describe you in the last two weeks.

YES	NO	**G** FMS General Characteristics **G**
		Widespread pain
		Above the waist
		Below the waist,
		Right side of the body
		Left side of the body
		Along the back and/or neck
		Abdomen and/or chest
		Fatigue
		Mental fatigue
		Physical fatigue
		Sleep disturbance
		Unable to get to sleep in 30 minutes or less
		Multiple awakenings # of awakenings/night_____
		Awaken feeling tired
		Interference with daily and work activities
		With daily self care activities. List_____
		With work activities. List_____
		With social/recreational activities. List_____

Other Associated Symptoms

YES	NO		YES	NO	
		Stiffness			PMS, disrupted
		Anxiety			menstrual cycle
		Memory problems			Clumsiness
		Irritable bowel			Restless leg syndrome
		syndrome			Cold hands, cold feet
		Irritable bladder			Pelvic pain
		syndrome			Jaw pain
		Headaches			Visual problems
		Dry mouth/eyes			Auditory problems
		Allergies			Sensory problems
		Numbness/tingling			Heart palpitations
		Swelling			Other_____

Symptom Pattern and Variation Questionnaire

Describe your symptoms.

- When do I feel the best?

    Days of the month? _____

    Days of the week? _____

    Times of the day? _____

    During or after what activities? _____

    After eating what foods/nutrients? _____

    Other _____

- When do I feel the worst?

    Days of the month? _____

    Days of the week? _____

    Times of the day? _____

    During or after what activities? _____

    After eating what foods? _____

    Other _____

- When I feel lousy what has helped relieve the symptoms?

    _____

    _____

    _____

    _____

My Results Summary

Insert results from pages 21 and 22.

General Characteristics I have:

1. _____

2. _____

3. _____

4. _____

5. _____

6. _____

Other associated symptoms I experience:

1. _____

2. _____

3. _____

4. _____

5. _____

6. _____

Symptom Patterns and Variations:

■ I feel the best _____

_____

■ I feel the worst _____

_____

■ I can help relieve symptoms by _____

_____

What Causes Fibromyalgia – What is going on?

Even though fibromyalgia has been documented for over 100 years in countries around the world, there has never been a definitive cause identified. In 1995 Yunus found indications for a genetic predisposition on chromosome six for fibromyalgia symptoms. Other research has shown that FMS is present in some family complexes and not in others. Research has discovered that FMS individuals can have alterations in several of the chemical messengers in their blood stream, spinal fluid, and urine as compared to normal controls. Most of these chemical assays are primarily performed in research labs and are not available in clinical situations. Research has also discovered that specific body systems are functioning abnormally in FMS. The systems found to be abnormal are the:

- hypothalamic-pituitary-adrenal axis
- autonomic nervous system axis, and
- reproductive hormone axis

Necklaces as Chemical Messengers

Chemical messengers maintain brain activity, they regulate mood, control sleep, appetite, memory, and mental alterness. Chemical messengers regulate muscle action, gut action, breathing patterns and heart rate. Chemical messengers determine energy levels, metabolic rate, and pain levels.

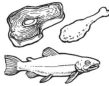

Most of the chemical messengers are formed from molecules of amino acids. The amino acids come from proteins.

When protein is eaten it is digested and broken into 20-30 different amino acids.

These different amino acids combine into chains – like necklaces. There are many combinations of amino acid chains just like there are many different kinds of necklaces. These chains of amino acids are called polypeptides. Familiar polypeptides include serotonin, enkephalins and insulin.

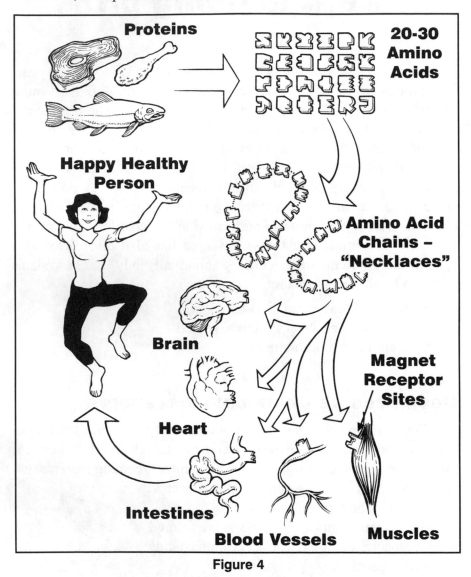

Figure 4

Manufacturing, Transporting, Receiving of Necklaces

The chemical messengers – amino acid chains – are manufactured at many sites throughout the body. They are manufactured in the brain, in glands like the thyroid, in organs like the pancreas and liver, in the digestive system, in the heart and ciruclatory system and in the muscles. A certain amino acid chain may be manufactured primarily at one site but will also have several other minor manufacturing "plants" at other sites. For example, 95% of the serotonin is produced in the gut but there are also manufacturing sites for serotonin in the brain and the muscles. Insulin is produced primarily in the pancreas but also in the brain and muscles.

These chemical messengers are transported via the blood stream or nerve fibers to many different receptor-magnet-sites where they regulate body functions. When they are present in nerve fibers they are known as neurotransmitters. When they are present in the blood stream they are known as hormones or biochemicals.

Receptor-magnet-sites for specific amino acid chains may be primarily on one organ or in one system but there will be multiple sites throughout the body with minor receptor-magnet-sites. For example, receptor-magnet-sites for serotonin are found in the pancreas, the intestines, the brain, and the heart. (Figure 4)

What Can Go Wrong with Necklaces?

The amino acid chains attached to receptor-magnet-sites activate and regulate organs and body systems that allow the human body and mind to function efficiently and without pain and fatigue. What can happen to alter this process?

- There may not be enough amino acid chains because of inadequate "raw materials" or precursors, i.e. proteins, vitamins, and minerals.
- There may be an inefficient manufacturing of protein to amino acid chains leading to excessive need for more and more protein and amino acids.

Chapter 3: What Causes Fibromyalgia? What Is Going On?

27

- There may be an excessive destruction of the chemical messengers before they have delivered the essential messages to the receptor-magnet-sites.
- There may be excessive production of the chemical messengers so they drown the receiving sites instead of providing important information on a gradual basis.
- The receptor sites may not be properly sensitive. The receptor-magnet-sites may not be powerful enough to attract and use the chemical messengers that arrive at the site.

Any disruption in the manufacturing, distribution, or use of these messengers results in body and mind dysfunction – pain, fatigue, memory problems, sleep disruption, sensory hypersensitivity, blood pressure changes, or digestive changes.

What Environmental Triggers Can Break the Necklaces?

Environmental triggers can set off FMS and are often described as "causing" FMS. A motor vehicle accident or a repetitive motion injury at work, a divorce, birth or death, a surgery, sexual abuse or an infection can act as the trigger that sets off the cascade of symptoms based on the underlying problem of the chemical messaging system. The body accommodates for the FMS, keeping the symptoms at a minimum, maintaining the balance within body functions until the trigger "upsets the applecart" as the saying goes. Once the trigger sets off the waterfall of symptoms it is difficult to reverse the process unless the underlying problem is understood.

Genetics and the Environment to Produce the Best Necklaces

We are ultimately products of our genetics and our environment. What happens in our lives triggers or inhibits genetic tendencies. If our genes predispose us to pain and fatigue we must minimize these tendencies through environmental interventions. This is no different than if genetics predispose an individual to be overweight. To minimize the genetic tendency for being overweight, increased exercise and decreased food intake is a necessity. In FMS the genetic tendency for disruption in the manufacturing, distribution, and/or use of amino acid messenger chains can be greatly exacerbated by environmental triggers. For FMS individuals to experienece minimal symptoms requires environmental modification – life style changes – to minimize the disruption in the messaging system.

Whose Job Is This Anyway?

The human body is regulated by control centers using the amino acid necklaces or fatty acid necklaces as chemical messengers. A disturbance in any one of these centers affects the other systems and the functioning of the human as a whole. Disturbances in three of these control systems have been identified in FMS individuals. The three systems are:

The Hypothalamic - Pituitary - Adrenal Axis (HPA)
The Autonomic Nervous System Axis (ANS)
The Reproductive Hormone Axis (RHA)

These three systems function independently to some extent but also influence each other on a regular basis. (Figure 5) Each system provides information and regulation to every cell in the body. Each system provides regulatory influence to the other two systems. Dysfunction in one system can influence dysregulation in the other two systems as well as disrupting body cellular function in general.

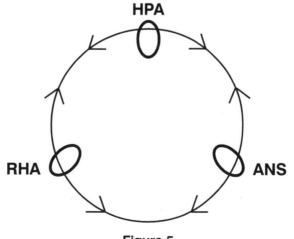

Figure 5

Chapter 3: What Causes Fibromyalgia? What Is Going On?

29

Hypothalamic · Pituitary · Adrenal (HPA) Axis

The Stress Axis

The hypothalamic - pituitary- adrenal axis is considered the stress system of the body because the chemical messengers given off by this combination of glands

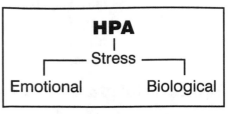

affect the body's ability to cope with stress, both emotional and biological. Biological stress includes dysfunction in metabolic and physiologic processes controlling blood pressure, blood sugar levels, and infection control, among other things. The hypothalamus, pituitary and adrenal glands produce chemical messengers that modulate pain, sleep, mood, sex drive, appetite, energy, and circulation.

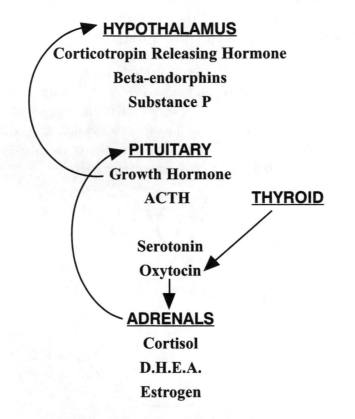

HYPOTHALAMUS

Corticotropin Releasing Hormone

Beta-endorphins

Substance P

PITUITARY

Growth Hormone

ACTH   **THYROID**

Serotonin

Oxytocin

ADRENALS

Cortisol

D.H.E.A.

Estrogen

Figure 6: HPA Axis Hormones

Many of the HPA axis hormones are found to be at abnormal levels in FMS. Serotonin is found in decreased amounts and Substance P is found in increased amounts in FMS individuals' cerebral spinal fluid. Growth hormone and cortisol are also found to be lower than normal in FMS. Dysfunction within the HPA axis can lead to fibromyalgia symptoms. When these chemical messengers are at abnormal levels the FMS individual experiences pain, sleep, mood, and energy changes.

The Autonomic Nervous System (ANS)

The autonomic nervous system is the control system sending messages from the brain to organs

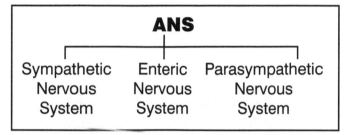

like the heart, lungs, intestines, bowel, and bladder. There are three subdivisions of the autonomic nervous system: the sympathetic, the parasympathetic and the enteric divisions. These are named for the locations from which they come. The sympathetic system comes from the thoracic and lumbar areas of the spine, the parasympathetic system comes from the cranial and sacral areas of the spine, and the enteric originates from the digestive system or gut. Contrary to popular belief, the sympathetic system is not always defined as excitatory, fight or flight, and the parasympathetic is not always quieting in nature. The sympathetic nervous system is slower and more widespread in its influence on the body systems. The parasympathetic nervous system is faster and more localized in its influence in the body. The parasympathetic nervous system action is more often restricted to a single organ while the sympathetic nervous system action more often affects the body as a whole. The enteric nervous system is the least known and understood division of the autonomic nervous system. It regulates intestinal or gut function.

The autonomic nervous system (ANS) and the HPA axis work together affecting each other and all other body systems. Norepinephrine (adrenaline) and neuropeptide Y produced in the ANS facilitate action in the HPA axis. Together the ANS and HPA axis influence areas of the brain involved in cognitive function, memory, memory retrieval and emotional analysis of experiences.

The Sympathetic and Parasympathetic Divisions

The heart, lungs, stomach, liver, pancreas, bladder, uterus, rectum and anus are all directed by sympathetic and parasympathetic divisions of the autonomic nervous system. When there is pain and dysfunction related to these organs, the autonomic nervous system will be involved in a direct or indirect way. There is most often an imbalance between the parasympathetic and sympathetic input to organ function. Excitatory, survival messages of the sympathetic system to organs become more predominant and enduring rather than a balance of excitatory and quieting directions that allow the organs to work and rest in a healthy rhythm. This imbalance in autonomic nervous system messaging and the resultant organ response leads initially to super efficient organ function at high energy levels. But as with any machine or body system, rest and maintenance is essential, and in this picture there is little or no rest/maintenance cycle. The result is an eventual melt down of organ function with the symptoms described by the individual as pain, fatigue, indigestion, diarrhea, shortness of breath and menstrual irregularity.

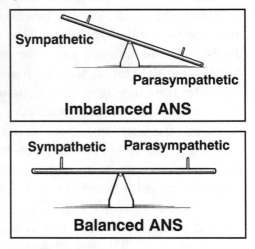

The muscles of the arms, legs, back and trunk are also influenced by the ANS. At rest these voluntary muscles have some tone/tension. The amount or degree of tone/tension present when the muscles are at rest is determined to a large extent by the sympathetic portion of the ANS. The muscle spindle functions much like a spring. The spring can be set tight or loose. If the spring is set tight the muscle has high resting tone. If the spring is set loose the muscle has low resting tone. The ANS sets the tightness or looseness of the spring. When the ANS is dysfunctional it will influence the muscles resulting in abnormally high resting tone. This affects the ability of muscles to work and rest efficiently and effectively.

Returning a balance to the sympathetic-parasympathetic divisions of the autonomic nervous system is essential in improving fibromyalgia symptoms.

The Enteric Division

An Electrical Messaging System

The enteric division of the autonomic nervous system is the gut's control system, the "gut's brain." It lines the digestive system from the esophagus to the anus. It is a vast chemical and electrical warehouse of messages that influence not only the digestive system but every other cell and organ system in the body. There are 100 million enteric nerves in the small intestine alone, more than in the entire peripheral nervous system and equal to the number in the spinal cord. The number of enteric nerves in the large intestine have yet to be counted. Only 1000-2000 nerve fibers connect the human brain to the enteric system through the vagus nerve. Therefore the gut's enteric nervous system functions on its own much more than it is directed by the human brain. We think of nerve messages as electrical events so it is easy to think of 2000 telephone lines between the head and gut compared to 100 million telephone lines within the small intestine. The 2000 messages sent from the head will be heard but the dominant voices will be from the enteric telephone system's electrical messages.

The enteric nervous system controls the efficiency and effectiveness of gut functions. The gut's major function is to digest food, absorb the digested nutrients into the blood stream and defend against poisons. The enteric nervous system determines to a large extent what nutrients and how much of each are absorbed or excreted.

A Chemical Messaging System

The enteric nervous system is a control system that sends its messages by chemicals as well as through electrical output. It produces information molecules that travel throughout the body to magnet sites on cells and organs. The same chemical messengers are produced by the enteric system and the brain. The "feel good" information molecules

– endorphins, the "pain perception" information molecules – substance P, the stress molecules – cortisol, and the calming information molecules – serotonin, are all produced in the gut's enteric nervous system and then travel to the rest of the body attaching to magnet sites and influencing function and behavior at that organ system site.

One of the most discussed information molecules in fibromyalgia is serotonin. Ninety five percent of the body's serotonin is produced in the gut not the brain! When the gut produces an abundance of serotonin it flows not only in the gut influencing function there but also to the head, to the heart, to the blood vessels, to the uterus, and to the bladder. What is serotonin's influence at the various sites? In the gut it facilitates contraction, in the heart it increases the heart rate, in the blood vessels it stimulates constriction, in the uterus and bladder it induces contraction, in the head it facilitates sleep and decreases pain perception.

Another chemical messenger produced by the enteric nervous system is substance P. Its influence is felt throughout the body. Substance P increases the perception of pain, it increases heart rate and decreases blood pressure.

When Humpty Dumpty Falls...

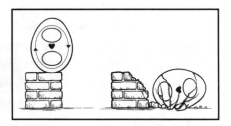

The enteric nervous system in fibromyalgia often has difficulty maintaining a balance between rest and work. One example is serotonin production by the enteric nervous system. The chemical messenger serotonin is released when there is pressure on the bowel lining cells. The serotonin excites peristalsis and thus elimination. If the release of serotonin is excessive then peristalsis is initially increased which causes diarrhea, dehydration and discomfort. As excessive serotonin production continues it "drowns" the gut's magnet receptor sites and as with any drowning victim the sites cease to function so the gut shuts down. This excessive serotonin results in paralysis of the gut until the excess serotonin is broken down or otherwise incapacitated. Constipation and even fecal impaction with inflammation results when the gut shuts down. Constipation and impaction of the gut is accompanied by abdominal pain, inability to stand up straight and a shuffling gait with quick fatigue. In severe cases the individual cannot get up from a chair without help.

Another example of imbalance in chemical messengers produced by the enteric nervous system is the production of substance P. Substance P excites pain fibers that travel to the brain with information about pain and discomfort. When excessive substance P is present in the gut and spinal fluid, pain messages increase along the pain fibers. Additionally, the fibers that transmit other sensations like touch, pressure, heat, cold, sound and light can become highly sensitized and begin to transmit messages that are interpreted by the brain as pain not just as touch, pressure or light sensation. Substance P has increased the body's pain sensitivity significantly without any major trauma having occurred.

An optimally functioning enteric division of the autonomic nervous system stimulates efficient function of the heart, lungs, uterus, bladder, brain, pancreas, liver, as well as the digestive system of the gut. When there is dysfunction or imbalance of the enteric system every other organ system is potentially dysfunctional as well. The enteric nervous system communicates with the heart via the vagus nerve complex, it communicates with the pancreas which produces insulin via enteric peripheral nerves and information chemicals, it communicates with uterus and bladder much the same way. If the enteric nervous system is in a high activation mode the gut will transfer food from mouth to anus faster than usual. Additionally the uterus and the bladder could be more irritable, the heart could beat faster, the pancreas could produce and dump increased amounts of insulin into the blood stream. The entire body is affected when the enteric nervous system of the gut is dysfunctional. The enteric nervous system and the gut become an essential focus of assessment and self care to manage fibromyalgia symptoms when the dysfunctional chemical and electrical messaging system is understood.

Who Is The Boss?

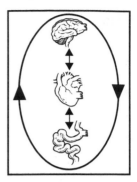

The head, heart and gut all have control centers described as both intrinsic and extrinsic. Intrinsic describes the ability to regulate their own organ system without external input. Extrinsic describes the ability to influence other organs and systems as well as their own. The ANS regulates the heart through the vagus nerve, a part of the parasympathetic division. The gut's enteric nervous system influences the heart through the same vagus nerve. This influence on the heart is significant but the heart also has its own intrinsic nervous system which keeps it functioning independent of outside control centers.

The heart will continue to beat in isolation just as the gut will continue to push food from the small intestine through the large intestine when there is no input from the human brain. Therefore symptoms of high heart rate, low blood pressure and abdominal pain are not necessarily mediated from the brain but rather may be influenced greatly by the heart's intrinsic control system "brain" and the gut's intrinsic control system (enteric) "brain."

The heart and gut's primary connection to the head is through the vagus nerve, an electrical messaging system. Messages from the brain to the heart and gut slows the heart rate and speeds up the gut peristalsis (rhythmical contractions). The enteric and cardiac control centers transmit messages to the brain via the vagus nerve informing and cajoling the brain centers in the head to provide necessary management of vital functions.

The heart, gut and head also communicate with each other via chemical messengers. These chemical messengers move through the blood stream to every cell of the body. When they find body cells that have receptors that attract them like magnets they attach and make significant changes in that cell structure and organ system. Therefore, in fibromyalgia the dysfunctional messaging systems can be both electrical and/or chemical.

In the past the treatment focus has been primarily to alter the brain's function. Now we begin to look at the possible dysfunction in the heart and gut because they too direct other body functions in a significant way. As Melissa, 21, said to her physician, "This condition is manic depression of the body not the mind." She was describing the erratic, unpredictable behavior of the gut and heart control centers that resulted in her pain, fatigue, and other FMS symptoms. To better explain the influence on the whole body, take the example of the lungs and breathing.

The Last Breath....

One of the major functions of the head, heart and gut control centers is to regulate the breathing diaphragm which is essential for life and health too. The breathing diaphragm functions under autonomic nervous system control most of the time to expand the lungs, filling them with oxygen and collapsing them to expel carbon dioxide. The breathing diaphragm does not have its own intrinsic nervous system so it cannot function in isolation from the head, heart and gut control centers. Rather it has dual innervation from the ANS and the voluntary nervous system. With ANS dysfunction, FMS individuals exhibit abnormal diaphragmatic breathing patterns. The breathing diaphragm action decreases and/or becomes shallow and ineffective. It is unable to automatically tighten and relax effectively, at times remaining in a semicontracted, tight state for long periods. This causes shortness of breath, chest, abdominal and back pain. Accessory muscles of the neck and upper chest take over much of the breathing activity but breathing effectiveness and efficiency is compromised. The internal organs, i.e., stomach, liver, pancreas, intestines, bladder, uterus and bowel are all suspended from the breathing diaphragm either directly or indirectly by fascial "strings" so that with every breath the breathing diaphragm takes the abdominal organs are gently, rhythmically moved. The gentle movement of the internal organs with each breath is significantly decreased when accessory muscles take over the breathing pattern. The breathing diaphragm is responsible for regulating the pH of every cell in the body – that is the acid-base balance of each cell. It regulates the carbon dioxide-oxygen balance throughout the body – essentially bringing needed oxygen to the cells and getting rid of waste carbon dioxide. The body pH changes with accessory muscle breathing compared to diaphragmatic breathing. Twelve to fourteen times per minute each minute of each day every day of the year the breathing diaphragm directed by the autonomic nervous system performs this essential function, or dysfunction as in the case of FMS. All of these changes can be precipitated by dysfunctional head, heart and gut control centers and lead to pain, fatigue, and associated symptoms of FMS.

The Reproductive Hormone Axis (RHA)

The Reproductive Hormone Axis includes the ovaries and uterus in females, the gonads in males, the adrenal glands and fat in females and males. Female and male chemical messengers are produced in these organs/glands in both males and females. The chemical messengers of the RHA are composed from fats broken down into essential fatty acids. Females will produce more female hormones than male hormones and vice versa but both females and males produce female and male hormones. Female hormones include estrogen, progesterone, relaxin, and oxytocin. The male hormone that is most familiar is testosterone.

Estrogen, Progesterone, and Testosterone

In females, estrogen and progesterone hormones (chemical messengers) produced primarily in the ovaries affect all organ systems including the brain, the gut, and the muscles. (Figure 7)

A consideration in FMS symptoms is the ratio of estrogen/progesterone to testosterone levels. Testosterone, the male hormone,

---

Female Reproductive Hormone Function

Estrogen	Progesterone
increases blood pressure	decreases blood pressure
improves sleep	decreases digestive activity
increases well being	increases appetite
increases energy	increases sex drive
increases endorphins	increases water retention
increases serotonins	increases breast engorgement
increases brain blood flow	decreases well being
increases thyroid function	

Figure 7

facilitates muscle definition and strength, modifies pain perception, and alters the distribution of fat around the waistline. An imbalance in the ratio of estrogen/progesterone to testosterone in females can aggravate muscle spasms and increase pain perception.

Daily, Monthly, Yearly Cycles

Estrogen and progesterone vary on a monthly/28 day cycle in the female. They also vary during the year, being at their highest level in April through July and being their lowest from October through January. When FMS individuals complain of increased symptoms during the winter months it may be that the estrogen/progesterone levels have fallen excessively much like the occurrence at the end of the monthly cycle. If increased symptoms occur in the spring it may be an over abundance of estrogen/progesterone. Supplementing with phyto-estrogens/progesterones in food or cream form or using hormone replacement therapy on a temporary or permanent basis may assist the organ systems in balanced function. In a clinical trial, pain and fatigue, bowel, bladder and menstrual cycle dysfunction improved in a small group of women who used phytoestrogen and progesterone during the winter months and again in the spring.

Mary described becoming incapacitated by Thanksgiving every year with pain, fatigue, abdominal bloating and gut dysfunction. She would be in bed, not be able to work or go to school. No dietary changes helped. She would gradually recover over a 4-6 week period. Using the phytoestrogen and progesterone creams she was able to work and attend school. She did not become ill or need to limit her activities any more than other times of the year. She states she has confidence that her life is under more control and balance.

Hormone levels vary on a daily cycle in males. It is typical for the levels to cycle up to eight times a day. Each of these cycles has the potential to affect FMS symptoms especially when there is an imbalance or variation in the cycle.

RHA-HPA-ANS
The Leg Bone is Connected to the Hip Bone...

The reproductive hormones help to regulate the HPA (hypothalamic-pituitary-adrenal axis) and vice versa. During chronic stress, there is a decrease in function of both the HPA and the RHA. Individuals under chronic stress exhibit diminished reproductive capability as well as fatigue, sleep disruption and illness. If there is a dysregulation of the RHA there will likely be an associated dysregulation of the HPA axis. For example, if estrogen, a part of the RHA, is chronically elevated, the HPA axis may well be significantly depressed. If RHA is in dysregulation the HPA opiods are decreased. Internally produced opiods are the natural analgesia in the body. Opioid receptors are present at all levels of the nervous system. Increased HPA axis dysregulation can increase the pain perception throughout the body. The ANS (autonomic nervous system) influences the HPA; the HPA influences the RHA; the RHA influences the ANS. The loop never ends and it can be affected at many junctions.

Chapter 4

How Is It Diagnosed? Who Has It?

Peggy R. Schlesinger, M.D.
Janet A. Hulme, P.T.

Fibromyalgia is often diagnosed using the 1990 American College of Rheumatology criteria of:

- Widespread pain of at least three months' duration.
- Pain to palpation at a minimum of 11 of the 18 tender point locations. The tender points are found throughout the body at specific sites (Figure 8). Tender points are areas of the body that are hypersensitive to pressure or touch. Tender points are painful and the FMS individual may flinch or unconsciously tighten the area when pressure is applied. In contrast, trigger points are hypersensitive areas of the body that, when pressure is applied, refer pain to a more distant body part as well as being painful over the site. Trigger points are present in myofascial pain syndrome.
- Associated symptoms often are present and include the 26 symptoms discussed in Chapter 1.
- A normal laboratory profile including complete blood count (CBC), sedimentation rate, antinuclear antibody, rheumatoid factor (RA), muscle enzymes, and thyroid function tests.

CBC measures levels of red, white and platelet cell numbers. Red blood cells store iron and a decrease in red blood cell numbers result in symptoms of fatigue. White blood cells fight infection. If they are decreased in number the immune system is impaired. Sedimentation rate (ESR) is the distance the blood cells fall in a test tube in one hour.

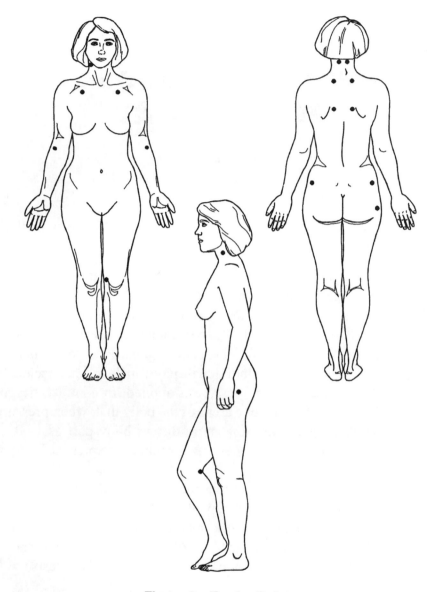

Figure 8 – Tender Points

With infection or inflammation they fall faster. Muscle enzyme tests eliminate the possibility of muscle diseases like muscular dystrophy. Thyroid function testing can pick up an under or overactive thyroid. Underactive thyroid can be associated with sore muscles and cold extremities in some individuals.

Blood tests are useful in ruling out possible diagnoses other than fibromyalgia even though they may accompany fibromyalgia as an additional diagnosis. These diagnoses include:

- Lyme disease
- Polymyalgia rheumatica
- Lupus erythematosus
- Hypothyroidism
- Inflammatory muscle diseases
- Giant cell arteritis
- Kawasaki's disease

Other possible differential or co-existing diagnoses include:

- Rheumatoid arthritis
- Parkinsonism
- Tendinitis
- Yeast infections

These may be present with FMS but the clinical diagnosis is more involved for these than any one specific lab test.

WHO HAS FIBROMYALGIA?

Approximately 1% of females between 20 and 30 years old have FMS. Up to 8% of individuals 70 and older experience FMS. There is a female to male ratio of eight or nine to two. The average age at the time of diagnosis is 49 but individuals describe having had symptoms for five or more years before diagnosis. The age range at diagnosis is six to 85 years old. Twenty-five percent have a childhood onset, 75% have adult onset. The onset is often insidious. Twenty percent of FMS occurs rapidly after surgery or trauma. Approximately 5 to 10% occurs following a febrile, usually a viral, illness. Twenty-five percent of FMS individuals have one or more other medical problems, i.e., degenerative joint disease, inflammatory arthritis, tendinitis, clinical depression, lupus erythematosus, or thyroid disease.

Even though FMS is described primarily in adults, children experience the same symptoms but are often undiagnosed or their symptoms overlooked. There is some indication that up to eight percent of the school population exhibit FMS symptoms. It is classified as juvenile primary fibromyalgia syndrome (JPFS). The criteria are:

- Presence of diffuse musculoskeletal aches, pains and stiffness for at least 3 months.
- Presence of at least ten typical and specific tender points.
- Symptoms modulated by such factors as weather, physical activity and anxiety/stress.
- Non-restorative sleep pattern.
- Absence of arthritic, inflammatory, endocrine or infectious cause for pain.

Children with FMS can complain of diffuse pain, stiffness, feeling of swelling, fatigue, poor sleep, waking tired, headaches, numbness/tingling, digestive problems, and anxiety.

Chapter 5

Does This Picture Of Fibromyalgia Fit Me?

Ellen S. Silverglat, M.S.W.
Erika Hulme
Janet A. Hulme, P.T.

Four individuals with fibromyalgia agreed to tell their unique stories. Each one experienced symptoms in his/her own way yet there is a similar thread throughout.

Fibromyalgia and Me, Adolescent Onset

My story of fibromyalgia is one of pain and confusion, as well as understanding, coping and solutions. I was diagnosed with fibromyalgia as a freshman in high school, but the pain preceded the diagnosis by many years. In fact, I cannot remember a time when I haven't had pain and headaches that often severely limited me.

My memories preceding my diagnosis are of confusion, loneliness and misunderstanding. I remember feeling confused about my pain because no one understood it or could figure out why I was in pain. I doubted my own feelings and often thought that maybe I was imagining it, that it wasn't real. I felt like a hypochondriac. Because of the pain and the confusion I never wanted to go out and play or be physically active. Instead, I read a lot and stayed in my room. Sometimes the only place I felt safe and comfortable was in my room and I would hide out there for hours. I felt out of place with other kids my age because all of them wanted to play sports and games that didn't interest me. I felt a push from everyone to do things out of doors and sometimes this would turn to anger when I wouldn't participate in the activities.

One of the hardest things for me was not knowing what was the matter. A part of me wanted to be out with my friends, just like a "normal" kid. Yet, I was always so tired and achy that I felt like I couldn't do anything. That part of me kept me down and there was always this conflict of interest.

I went to doctor after doctor for specific problems that I would later learn all stemmed from the fibromyalgia. I went to a specialist for knee pain and my family practitioner for stomach pain several times. Nothing was ever completely explained. The final event that led to a diagnosis was shoulder pain that prevented me from lifting my arm over my head. A rheumatologist finally diagnosed my fibromyalgia at the end of my freshman year in high school.

Of course, the pain did not disappear following the diagnosis. Knowing what I had was still just the first step in understanding and coping with the pain I had been experiencing. In high school there were two periods of time when I felt so bad that I didn't go to school for days at a time. My stomach always hurt and I felt like all I could do was lie in bed and sleep. I guess I was kind of depressed, but at the time I wouldn't have described it that way. It was more just an exhaustion dragging me down and making me not want to get out of bed. Both times I only got better with a lot of encouragement from my mother. She made me get out of bed and do some walking and other daily activities that I would have neglected. Finally, I would start to feel better and slowly get back into my old life and activities.

There have been many obstacles to overcome in living with fibromyalgia. One of the toughest has been dealing with people. It is really difficult explaining to friends what is the matter with me and how it limits my life. I can't just say "I broke my arm" or "I have mono." People understand those limitations and can respond to them. Fibromyalgia requires much more explaining and I don't even totally understand it, so how do I try to explain something I don't comprehend? Family members come to understand enough to get by, but even they don't really know what it is like or how it affects everything I do.

Friends are harder to deal with. They want you to be fun and active with them all the time. It has been even harder with my teachers. Usually I don't even try to explain it to them because when I have tried I have gotten blank stares. They say they understand and then it is pushed into the recesses of their minds or completely forgotten.

I've been on and off different medications since my diagnosis. I've found that I am sensitive to most medication so a majority of the time I cope with the pain without medication. I took one medication for a little over half a year until I had an adverse reaction to it. It lowered my blood pressure and raised my heart rate causing dizziness and faintness. I then tried another medication, but had a terrible reaction that caused cold sores and a skin rash.

The thing I hate most is the limits that fibromyalgia places on my life. I always have to think before I participate in any activity that I know might end up making me miserable the next day. The repercussions my actions might have on my body always have to be a major concern. The hardest thing for me is putting myself first, no matter what I have to put aside to do it, even if it is studying for an exam or not going out with friends. I have found that if I am the priority I can do more and the pain actually interferes less with my life. I still go out and have fun with my friends, and still get good grades. I just have to plan better and make the most of the times that I feel good.

It has taken a long time to acknowledge and respond quickly to the clues my body gives me that help me deal with this on a daily basis. I've learned that if I am feeling grouchy or feel myself getting annoyed easily with everything I need to think about what is really bothering me. Usually it is a headache and I now know that I need to lie down and relax to help it go away. To help care for myself I take a little time each day by myself to just relax and not think about anything. This time helps me to focus on being quiet and calm. I also try to have fun each day, no matter how much I have to do.

It goes without saying that growing up with fibromyalgia has affected my life. I can look back and see that the reason I stayed inside and read rather than playing games with my friends was probably because I was hurting or had a headache. In some ways I think I missed out on a lot, but I am also a stronger person. I am much more aware of my limits and abilities.

Right now I am a senior in college. Some days are bad, but for the most part I feel good and am able to be a successful student. I know that I am very fortunate to be doing as well as I am and that I am able to lead what is for the most part a normal life. It isn't easy, but I manage. I think that is the key word for people with fibromyalgia, MANAGEMENT.

A WOMAN'S STORY

I have been asked to share my story about living with fibromyalgia. Boy that sounds dramatic to me, because I don't think I live differently than anyone else . . . denial? most likely. Let me tell you a little about myself. I am almost 30 years old. I grew up in Europe, was raised by successful and supportive parents. My mom never ran out of energy, but I do remember her being in pain . . . and she still is. I am the oldest of three children. As a young child I was very physically active but I often complained of pain. I think my mom thought I was "getting hurt" and suggested I start swimming. What a great idea! I love to swim. I swam competitively in high school and college and was ranked at a national and international level.

I now know that I have fibromyalgia. I had to be very persistent with my doctors to have them look at fibromyalgia as the possible cause of my problems. I complained of some part of my body aching or hurting every day and swallowed up to 20 Advil a day. I didn't realize other people didn't hurt like this. I had chest pain and shortness of breath. I experienced vision problems but the glasses they prescribed did not help. I felt fatigued a lot. The physician said it was normal to be tired with all the swimming I did, but none of my friends were as worn down as I was and some even swam longer distances. I had "tendinitis" of every tendon possible which was treated with ice (which I hated) and antiinflammatory drugs. The things I never complained of because I didn't want to be labeled as crazy included: transient concentration problems, inability to eat certain foods, irritability, mood swings, extreme abdominal pains, bowel problems, inability to cope with noises and inability to be rational when I was tired. Associated with the fibromyalgia, I had heart problems diagnosed as idiopathic arrhythmia in 1993. Initially I was unable to climb a flight of stairs without multiple rests. I was experiencing angina just sitting around. Eventually I found a cardiologist who worked with me and encouraged my athletics again.

Today I am the director of physical therapy at a major urban hospital. I am also enrolled in an MBA program on a part-time basis and guest lecture at a local physical therapy school. I compete in master's swimming and in triathlons. To do this I must take care of myself in very specific ways. I avoid extreme temperature changes. I have to acclimate to altitude slowly. I avoid extreme emotional situations and stresses when possible. I prevent hypoglycemic attacks by eating frequent and regular small meals. I have to get 8-10 hours sleep a night. I take medication and vitamins regularly. I avoid caffeine and drink plenty of liquid. I accept my fatigue days and limit my activities on those days.

It is wonderful to have many good days and to be able to effectively treat the bad days. My husband is a big reason for me to finally get the proper care. He laughs with me when I tell him my hair hurts. I know that getting frustrated and angry only makes me worse (that doesn't mean I don't get frustrated and angry at times). I feel healthy. I still have big dreams. My biggest dream is to finish the Iron Man Triathlon in Hawaii. Some people would say that my "plate" is full. Yes, it is and I don't know it to be different.

A SECOND WOMAN'S STORY

About five years ago I noticed a tremor in my left hand and that my fingertips were turning white at times. Then my leg muscles started twitching, sometimes making my whole leg move, especially at night. I felt very tired and I had periodic diarrhea so I thought I had the flu but it never went away. Over several months the tremors in my arms and legs decreased but the aching in my neck and back was so much that I couldn't sit at my desk and work for more than two hours, and that exhausted me for the rest of the day. I quit my job four years ago and have not been able to work since then.

There are some days now that I can get up, take my shower, get dressed and do some light housework before noon. After doing this I have to rest for at least two hours in the afternoon so I have enough energy to fix something easy for dinner by 5:00 p.m. Then at night I watch TV or play cards with my husband, but it even hurts to hold the cards in my hands some nights. On bad days I am in bed most of the day because I hurt and have no energy.

I have been to at least a dozen different doctors and tried every medication in the book, but I have severe side effects to most of the ones I've tried and the others haven't helped. I am better than I was four years ago and I plan to start a typing service in my home so I can work at my own pace. I have always liked to work and just one or two hours a day will be better than nothing.

A MAN'S STORY

I am a construction worker and injured my right shoulder two years ago pulling cable. It was diagnosed as a rotator cuff injury. I had physical therapy and finally surgery one year ago. When I went back to work I felt pain in both shoulders and into my back and neck. My right hand started going numb when I drove truck or pulled cable. I have a high tolerance for pain but work tired me out so much that when I got home I was out of sorts and went to bed early.

Even though I went to bed early I woke in the morning feeling terrible. Sometimes I woke up ten times during the night. It took me until noon to work out all the kinks. I felt like Frankenstein in the morning, feeling very stiff and moving awkwardly. By afternoon I could bend and reach more easily.

I used to work out in the gym and lap swim 3-4 nights a week after work. I hated to admit it but I was too tired and sore to do it. If I went twice a month I was lucky. My two sons complained that I wouldn't play baseball with them but when I pitched more than a half dozen balls I started to get a headache and my back and shoulder started hurting. My family life had really gone downhill. I slept on the couch half the time because I was so restless and up so many times my wife said she couldn't sleep. I pushed through the pain but my family said they didn't know me anymore and they saw what the pain was doing to me more than I did. I guess I just got used to it and forgot about what I used to be like.

Six months later.

I am doing a lot better now. I started on medication six months ago and also learned some biofeedback and pacing techniques. I had six weeks more physical therapy tailored more for fibromyalgia than a shoulder injury. We do some of the physical therapy at home when I have more pain than usual. I am continuing to work and now I work out 2-3 days a week at the gym and swim or walk the other days. I sleep well most nights and don't feel like a zombie when I wake up. However, I still take a hot shower and loosen up first thing in the morning. My boys say I can throw the ball better and I'm more fun to be around. My wife says I still don't do enough around the house when I get home but she will put up with it to have her husband back.

PART II - WHO CAN HELP?

Chapter 6

What Can Physicians Do To Help?

Peggy Schlesinger, M.D.
Muriel R. Friedman, M.D.
Barbara Penner, P.T.
Janet A. Hulme, P.T.

A physician who knows about fibromyalgia is the keystone of an effective team which includes the individual, family members, other medical and complementary care personnel, friends and relatives, and work acquaintances. Most frequently the physician is an internist, a family practice physician, a physiatrist, or a rheumatologist. Essential aspects of a health care team are: knowledge, interest, and the concept of a wellness model for chronic care.

The physician will take a complete history of present and past problems. He/she will review the results of blood tests and X-rays as well as results of special tests used to eliminate other illnesses which could cause the same symptoms. The physician will perform a physical exam which includes palpation of tender points and assessment of functional movement of neck, back, arms and legs. The diagnosis of fibromyalgia is made from the results of the evaluation.

Once the diagnosis is made, the physician recommends appropriate medications and follows up on the patient's response to treatment and evaluates side effects if any. The physician coordinates the health care team in developing treatment strategies. Treatment strategies include techniques for pain relief, sleep disturbance relief, daily self care management, self care crisis management, and quality of life restoration which may hopefully include a return to work and full function. Fibromyalgia is not a curable problem so the physician's ultimate role is to assist the individual in taking control of his/her illness, taking over self care for pain, fatigue, and other symptoms. The physician assists the individual in knowing when and how the medical team can help.

Rheumatologist

A rheumatologist is a specialist in painful conditions affecting joints and the connective tissue, fascia, muscles and tendons of the body. Rheumatology is a specialized branch of internal medicine whose role it is to tease out difficult diagnostic problems affecting adults, especially when they involve pain in and around joint structures. For many rheumatologists as much as one third of their practice involves caring for FMS individuals. Besides determining the appropriate diagnosis, the rheumatologist coordinates and prioritizes the services provided by the rest of the health care team.

Some physician specialists become involved with FMS individuals for associated problems of fibromyalgia. Those may include a urologist, an obstetrician-gynecologist, an orthopedic surgeon, and a neurologist.

Urologist

Urologists diagnose and treat bladder problems. Since fibromyalgia affects smooth muscle and circulation in the bladder, symptoms of urgency, frequent urination, enuresis (uncontrolled leaking of urine), lower abdominal discomfort and flank or kidney pain in the absence of test findings of infection, obstruction or tumors can often be linked to fibromyalgia. When the symptoms are chronic (1-2 years) and include frequent urination (multiple times an hour during the day and more than two times at night), feeling the urge to urinate but having very little flow, a bloated feeling of discomfort/pain in the lower abdomen, the diagnosis may be interstitial cystitis, fibromyalgia, or a combination of the two. Urethral syndrome symptoms (frequent urination and discomfort with urination) can be caused by fibromyalgia. FMS is usually not the primary cause of incontinence but it can be a significant contributing factor such that until the FMS is treated appropriately the incontinence symptoms will persist at least periodically. Fibromyalgia can be involved in urge, mixed and enuresis types of incontinence much more than stress incontinence (leaking with jumping, running or coughing). Since FMS symptoms include bladder and bowel symptoms, the effective treatment of FMS often significantly reduces the bladder and bowel symptoms. If the symptoms persist after the FMS has improved, a referral to a urologist is recommended. Urologists can then perform special tests and recommend treatment for the specific bladder or bowel condition. In all the urological disorders mentioned, treatment includes medication and reeducation of the pelvic muscles, bladder, and abdominal muscles via exercise, massage, and physiological quieting.

Orthopedic Surgeon

An orthopedist is a surgeon who operates on bones and joints. When multiple symptoms coexist with the core FMS symptoms many individuals think there may be more than one diagnosis. Symptoms such as numbness and tingling or shooting pain can bring about concern that other problems such as tendinitis, bursitis, thoracic outlet syndrome, carpal tunnel syndrome, ulnar nerve compression, and even sciatica may be playing a role. Because FMS can be associated with all these myriad symptoms it is advisable to treat the FMS first and see how well the other symptoms respond. Many times the other problems are resolved with general FMS treatment. An orthopedic surgeon is consulted if unusual symptoms persist. An orthopedic surgeon who is familiar with fibromyalgia will ask the key questions, evaluate, and treat for the specific orthopedic problem.

Obstetrician-Gynecologist

Abdominal and pelvic pain can be a predominant symptom for some FMS individuals. An obstetrician/ gynecologist and gastroenterologist may be involved in differentiating the symptoms of tumors and infections of the reproductive organs and intestines from fibromyalgia. During pregnancy, the biomechanical and hormonal changes may increase back pain, thoracic outlet syndrome or carpal tunnel symptoms. When the obstetrician is aware the individual has FMS, the care can be specialized to provide for optimum comfort and function. Increased pain symptoms respond well to treatments such as gentle exercise, massage, heat and modalities.

Neurologist

A neurologist evaluates and treats dysfunction of the nervous system. Diagnostic tests are performed to rule out diseases of the nervous system such as multiple sclerosis, Parkinson's disease or amyotrophic lateral sclerosis. A neurologist performs nerve conduction velocity tests to determine if the pain, numbness, and tingling the individual describes is a nerve compression problem such as carpal tunnel syndrome or ulnar nerve compression.

Where there is another diagnosis in conjunction with fibromyalgia, treating the fibromyalgia first, then seeing what symptoms remain has been the most effective approach. It is advisable that any physician a FMS individual chooses should have a working knowledge of fibromyalgia and its implications.

As one FMS individual said about finding a doctor. "I have looked long and hard for my doctor. The one I have now listens, always gives me options for treatment, involves my family, and encourages me to be independent and try new things. He is wonderful about keeping up on new medications that might help."

Chapter 7

What Medications Can Help?

Janet A. Hulme, P.T.
Gayle Cochran, Pharm.D.

Drug treatments will help some individuals and not others. Some medications act immediately while some take weeks or months to have an effect. Some medications become less effective with long term use so a different medication must be tried. At some point in fibromyalgia treatment medications are often used on a trial and error basis to find which ones are most effective to relieve the individual's symptoms and have the fewest side effects. It is important to take the medication over the long term, not just when symptoms are present. Like a diabetic, there is a chemical imbalance or lack of certain chemicals needed for health, and the medication is needed on a regular basis to best maintain symptom relief.

Summary of Symptom Relief Medications

Anxiety - Benzodiazepines

Sleep Disturbance - Tricyclic antidepressants, Benzodiazepines, Calcium, Melatonin, Valerian

Fatigue - Selective serotonin reuptake inhibitors (SSRI)

Irritable Bowel Syndrome - Antispasmodics (Bentyl, Levsin), Tricyclic antidepressants, Imodium, Magnesium, Vitamin C, Dietary Fiber

Irritable Bowel Syndrome - Tricyclic antidepressants, Urised

Headaches - Nonsteroidal anti-inflammatories, Calcium channel blockers, Imitrex

Restless Leg Syndrome - Sinemet, Klonopin, Vitamin E, Calcium and Magnesium combined

Descriptions of Commonly Used Medications

Tricyclic Antidepressants (TCA)

Function: Increase CNS neurotransmitter levels (serotonin and/or norepinephrine)
Effect: Sedation, diminish fatigue, decrease pain, elevate mood
Dose: 5-75 mg often at bedtime - dose varies with drug
Side Effects: Racing heart, nightmares, hangover, sedation, dry mouth, urinary retention, constipation
Examples: amitriptyline (Elavil)
nortriptyline (Pamelor)
doxepin (Sinequan)
desipramine (Norpramin)

Cyclobenzaprine (Flexeril)

A tricyclic amine, it is a muscle relaxant.

Nefazadone (Serzone)

Function: Inhibits uptake of serotonin and norepinephrine
Effect: Decrease pain, diminish fatigue
Side Effects: Nausea, headaches, postural hypotension
Note: Not to be taken with monoamine oxidase inhibitors

Nonsteroidal Anti-Inflammatories – (NSAIDs)

Function: Inhibits prostaglandin synthesis

Effect: Blocks pain and inflammation at local tissue level

Dose: 600-800 mg/day for analgesic level

Side Effects: Nausca, stomach pain, ulcers, fluid retention, renal toxicity in older individuals

Examples: ibuprofen (Motrin, Advil),
naproxen (Naprosyn, Aleve)

Benzodiazepines

Function: Increase GABA (gamma aminobutryric acid) which acts on thalamus to inhibit anxiety

Effect: Diminish pain and anxiety, increase sleep

Dose: Varies with particular agent

Side Effects: Sedation, depression

Examples: alprazolam (Xanax)
clonazepam (Klonopin)

Note: Dependency/addictive qualities

Tramadol (Ultram)

Function: Increases serotonin and norepinephrine, increases opioid reception; a synthetic analgesic

Effect: Inhibits pain perception, decreases pain

Dose: 50 mg, 2-4/day

Side Effects: Dizziness, nausea, constipation, headaches, postural hypotension

Note: Dependency/addictive qualities

Zolpidem (Ambien)

Function: Non-benzodiazepine sedative/hypnotic

Effect: Increased duration of sleep, decreased time to get to sleep

Dose: 5-10 mg

Side Effects: Memory problems, daytime drowsiness, dizziness, headache, nausea

Note: Short term treatment of insomnia only, 7-10 days, dependency/addictive qualities

Serotonin Reuptake Inhibitors
Function: Blocks destruction of serotonin so its effects last longer (controls food intake, temperature regulation, anxiety)
Effect: Diminish pain, fatigue, and anxiety; improve mood
Dose: 20-200mg depending on agent
Side Effects: Anxiety, nervousness, insomnia, tremor, dizziness
Examples: fluoxetine (Prozac)
sertraline (Zoloft)
paroxetine (Paxil)
venafaxine (Effexor)

Calcium Channel Blockers
Function: Dilates arteries, lowers blood pressure, inhibits contraction of smooth vascular muscle, especially of the cerebral arteries
Effect: Decrease pain, headaches, fatigue, memory problems; improves circulation
Dose: Up to 30 mg 2-3 times a day or once daily slow release 60 mg (depends on drug)
Side Effects: Decreased blood pressure, flushing, swelling in feet, constipation, dizziness
Examples: nimodipine (Nimotop) 30 mg
diltiazem 60-240 mg (many strengths and trade names)

Vasodilators
Function: Vasodilation of arteries or veins
Effect: (Experimental in nature) diminish pain, fatigue, anxiety, memory deficits
Dose: Varies with agent
Side Effects: Light headedness, headaches, tachycardia reflex
Examples: Nitroglycerin 0.4 mg sublingual
Hydralazine 25 mg

Estrogen Replacement Therapy
Can stabilize hormonal levels in females, may improve cognitive function and improve vasomotor stability.

Growth Hormone

Nutropin: At this time experimental only; release stimulated by serotonin and dopamine.

Combination Therapies

- **Prozac** and **Sinequan**
  Restlessness caused by Prozac balanced by Sinequan quieting
- **Prozac** and **Elavil**
  Elavil at night restores normal sleep pattern and Prozac in the morning helps decrease morning drowsiness.
- **Klonopin** and **Sinequan**
  Klonopin gets you to sleep, Sinequan keeps you there
- **Xanax** and **NSAID** (Motrin) antianxiety, analgesia

Note: Any sedating antidepressant at bedtime may be used with any of the SSRIs in the morning, for example trazadone (Desyrel), a sedative, used with sertraline (Zoloft), an SSRI.

Trigger Point Injections

Trigger points, when pressure is applied to the area, are painful at the site and refer pain to other areas of the body. They are a sign of a myofascial pain pattern or syndrome. Tender points are exquisitely painful at the site of pressure only and are a sign of fibromyalgia.

Injections into trigger points in FMS are appropriate if there is also myofascial pain in conjunction with FMS symptoms. The trigger points are injected with:

- Lidocaine, procaine (local anesthetics)
- Cortisone – in small amounts, less frequently. There may be increased pain for up to 48 hours after the injection, then there should be a decrease in pain over the long term. Systemic side effects almost never occur if the volume injected is below 5 cc, but this is dependent on the potency of the steroid.

Antiyeast Regimens

- Lactobacillus Acidophilus
- Co Enzyme Q
- Vitamin B 12
- Fluconazole for 1-3 weeks, Nystatin as maintenance

Local Anesthetic Sprays / Oils / Creams

- Vapocoolant spray – see Chapter 12
- Topical creams
  trolamine salicylate 10% (Myoflex)
  capsaicin (Zostrix) cream decreases pain by decreasing
  substance P
- Essential Oils – see Chapter 12

Nutritional

- Vitamin C 500-1,000 mg
- Vitamin B Complex 25-50 mg
- Vitamin E 200-400 IU
- Magnesium 500-800 mg
- Calcium 1000-1500 mg
- Malic Acid 1200-1400 mg

Herbal / Natural Products

- Licorice – Use natural not synthetic form. Used to increase blood volume and increase low blood pressure in vasopressor syncope.
- Melatonin – Secreted by pineal gland and made from serotonin. It helps set the sleep/wake cycle.
- Valerian – Used to treat sleep disturbance.
- Echinacea – Used to decrease pain.
- Calms Forte – Used to improve sleep and anxiety.
- Rhus Toxicodendron – Used to treat stiffness.
- Ginger – Used to improve irritable bowel syndrome.
- Cayenne – Used to improve circulation and digestion, to decrease pain.

- Peppermint – Used to improve digestion and decrease intestinal cramping.
- Chamomile – Used to improve sleep and decrease intestinal cramping.

Note: herbals are not FDA controlled.

More details about nutrition are available in Chapter 12.

Medications for Juvenile Fibromyalgia Syndrome

These include cyclobenzaprine, amytriptyline, and trazodone. Before adolescence, education and biofeedback are recommended initially and medication is used only if the education and biofeedback are not adequate.

Chapter 8

What Can Traditional And Alternative Medicine Do To Help?

Janet A. Hulme, P.T.
Gail E. Nevin, P.T.

Traditional and alternative health care offer beneficial interventions in managing FMS. These interventions are helpful in decreasing pain, fatigue, and sleep disturbance, as well as increasing endurance in daily activities and work. Traditional and alternative health care can include the techniques and modalities of physical and occupational therapy, chiropractic therapy, massage therapy, acupressure, acupuncture, and naturopathy.

Heat

Pain control is often the first priority. Heat in the form of hot packs and heating pads, and hot water in the form of hot tubs, hot showers or whirlpools, decreases pain by increasing circulation and relaxing muscle and joint structures. Cold is also used at times for pain control. Crushed ice, cold packs, and ice cups produce numbness and decreased pain. A combination of heat and cold alternating every 5-7 minutes for 20 minutes may be beneficial. Vapocoolant spray and heat is also used to decrease pain.

Ultrasound therapy is helpful at times. High frequency sound waves are transmitted from the head of the equipment to the muscles, ligaments and fascia through a thin film of conductive gel. Ultrasound waves cause vibration of muscle cells increasing circulation and relaxing muscle tightness. Ultrasound is often effective at .5-.75 watts per centimeter squared, pulsed for 3-5 minutes.

Electrical Modalities

Equipment using electrical current may assist in pain control for fibromyalgia. Equipment that can be helpful includes high voltage galvanic stimulation, interferential current stimulation, and microamperage stimulation. Electrical current in the various forms increases circulation and facilitates muscle relaxation as well as decreases pain. Electrical stimulation is delivered through moist pads placed over muscle areas which are connected to a piece of equipment via wires. The electric stimulation causes pulsation and a "buzzing" may be felt during the treatment. High voltage galvanic stimulation is often effective at 50-100 volts, 80 pulses per second, negative polarity, 2.5 seconds reciprocal for 20 minutes. Microamperage is often effective at .5 uv for 20 minutes using silver-silver chloride electrodes.

Physiological Quieting

Physiological Quieting (PQ) assists in decreasing pain levels and improving sleep quality and quantity. PQ includes diaphragmatic breathing, handwarming and body-mind quieting. PQ normalizes autonomic nervous system function, balances the communication between the head brain and the gut brain (enteric nervous system), and balances the communication from the body to the brain with the brain messages to the body. Hourly handwarming and diaphragmatic breathing for 30 seconds at a time and nightly use of the PQ audiotape is often effective in significantly improving sleep and decreasing pain. See Chapter 12 for an in-depth discussion of Physiological Quieting.

Exercise

As pain, fatigue, and sleep disturbance improve, strength and endurance becomes a priority. Progressive exercise programs for joint and muscle flexibility, muscle strength, and cardiovascular (heart and lung) fitness are priorities. Range of motion and stretching exercises decrease stiffness and improve flexibility. Vapocoolant spray and heat can often increase flexibility while decreasing pain and stiffness (see Chapter 12). Isometric (pushing against an immovable object), isokinetic or isotonic (moving an arm or leg through space) exercise increases muscle strength. Cardiovascular fitness through aerobic exercise means gradually increasing the strength of the heart, lungs, and circulation. Walking, biking, or swimming for 20-30 minutes daily is recommended.

Exercise is often accomplished with less pain and faster progression if done in a warm pool (see Chapter 20). Water at shoulder height significantly decreases the effect of gravity on an individual's body. There is a feeling of weightlessness. A warm pool (85-92°F) increases circulation and improves muscle relaxation. Using a hot tub before and after exercise is also helpful.

Endurance in daily activities improves as strength and flexibility increases. Tasks include developing daily pacing, energy conservation, work/rest cycles and fun/work cycles in conjunction with the vocational goals of the individual. Altering daily tasks such as dressing, cooking, driving, writing, and telephoning, so that they are efficient and pain free is essential. Assistance in maintaining job tasks through ergonomic and equipment changes and scheduling modifications enables pain free long term employment.

Over months and years, reevaluations by a professional provide tracking of the individual's progress so he/she knows there is improvement, that there is improvement even though the steps taken are small and there are setbacks along the way. Health care professionals provide reinforcement in terms of learning to manage while continuing to try new skills and experiences.

Massage Therapy

Massage can be helpful for pain relief, improved circulation, relaxation of muscles and removal of waste product build up. Massage needs to start gently; pain is not gain in fibromyalgia. As the muscles release, deeper massage may be appropriate. Special techniques, including craniosacral and myofascial release techniques, can be appropriate and beneficial. Massage therapists, physical therapists, occupational therapists, nurses, and chiropractors are all individuals trained in massage.

For self massage, balls, theracane, even the sharp corner of a wall can be used to assist with pressure techniques. Tender point pressure and acupressure, as well as relaxation massage techniques, can be learned by the individual and a supportive family member. Using essential oils with massage may bring additional pain relief.

Manipulation Therapy

Manipulations and adjustments of joints to properly align the vertebra or other body segments can be beneficial in decreasing the pain and muscle tension and increasing circulation and nerve flow for fibromyalgia individuals. Spinal alignment is temporary if muscle tightness and spasm alters vertebral position. Osteopathic physicians, chiropractic physicians, and physical therapists are trained in this area of treatment.

Acupressure / Acupuncture Therapy

Acupressure and acupuncture are non-medicinal ways to help control pain. Acupressure uses pressure rather than needles to treat key areas of the body. Acupressure can be performed by the individual or a friend by applying pressure with the middle finger or thumb to acupressure points. A physical therapist, massage therapist, chiropractor or physician may have the training for acupressure treatment.

Acupuncture is a form of Chinese medicine in which inserting fine needles into the skin of the ear, the feet or other body parts relieves chronic pain, fatigue or other neurological symptoms. Pain relieving brain chemicals called endorphins and enkephalins are released during acupuncture. These chemicals block the pain circuits from sending their message to the brain so "you don't feel the pain." Acupuncture has few side effects if disposable, standard needles are used and are administered by a trained acupuncturist. Pain relief should be felt within 5-10 treatments. Acupuncture can be used to improve the associated symptom related to FMS as well as the pain. Treating the Chinese organs or meridians of spleen, liver, kidney, lung and heart through acupuncture can be beneficial in relieving FMS symptoms. Physician acupuncturists and licensed acupuncturists are qualified to administer this treatment.

Naturopathic Medicine

Naturopathic medicine focuses on facilitating the body's innate healing abilities through use of natural medicines which support the body and work in conjunction with the immune system to restore health. Naturopathic medicine addresses the physical, mental, and emotional aspects of dysfunction. Treatment possibilities include nutritional analysis, dietary alterations, constitutional homeopathic remedies, botanical medicines, hormone therapy, counseling and hydrotherapy. Nutritional analysis includes food intake, digestive capacity, and elimination patterns. Dietary recommendations may include foods to avoid such as coffee, chocolate, vinegar, pickled foods, acidic plant foods, alcohol, carbonated drinks, shellfish, white sugar, white flour, artificial additives and preservatives, and processed foods. A detoxification diet is often recommended. Supplementation can include omega 3 and 6 fatty acids and multiple vitamins. Constitutional homeopathy can include an individually prescribed remedy to address symptoms and susceptibility of the immune system. Botanical medicines are used to affect inflammation, liver function, the digestive system, nervous system, endocrine and circulatory systems. Hormone therapy can include DHEA, melatonin and phytoestrogen and progesterone. Hydrotherapy includes herbal, Epsom salts, and mineral baths.

Magnet Therapy

The use of magnets to relieve pain has been beneficial for some FMS individuals. Magnets are imbedded in shoe insoles, belts, bracelets, mattress pads, or taped over areas of pain. Our body systems are electromagnetic in nature and all of the implications involving use of magnets are poorly understood at this time.

What Can A Pain Clinic Do To Help?

In certain situations an inpatient or outpatient pain clinic may be an appropriate treatment approach. A team approach with the patient and his/her family as the center includes medical specialities of physical therapy, occupational therapy, vocational rehabilitation, psychology, nutrition, and physician. The goal is to enable the individual to return to daily activities of self care, family interaction, social interaction and to the vocational/work situation. The effective pain clinic works within the individual's limits, to develop coping skills, to develop and implement self care skills for pain and fatigue and to prescribe appropriate nonaddictive medications. Appropriate medications can enable the FMS individual to increase his/her endurance, strength, and daily activities initially in a controlled environment, then on an independent basis in society.

A typical daily routine in a pain clinic modified for the FMS individual might be:

8:00 a.m.	hot shower and gentle stretching, breakfast
9:00 a.m.	physiological quieting
9:30 a.m.	stretching with breathing; overall body strengthening using theraband
10:15 a.m.	rest cycle with biofeedback, snack
10:30 a.m.	lifting, carrying, standing, sitting tolerance, vocational skill modification
11:30 a.m.	rest cycle with quieting music
11:45 a.m.	lunch with nutritional education
1:00 p.m.	aerobic pool exercise or stationary bike or treadmill stretches in hot tub
2:00 p.m.	group therapy, behavior modification
3:15 p.m.	rest period, snack
3:30 p.m.	physical therapy modalities, massage
4:15 p.m.	structured leisure activities
5:00 p.m.	dinner

Initial evaluation and goal setting by the interdisciplinary team and weekly reassessment individualizes the treatment schedule. The questions are:

- What activities can I do and still have tolerable pain levels?
- What skills can help me with pain and fatigue?
- What medications can help?
- How can I approach work, home, family and leisure activities in a healthy way?
- How can I learn to rest effectively at night and throughout the day?
- How can I float through life's activities and stressors instead of being the bull in a china closet?

Chapter 9

What Can Biofeedback Do To Help?

Gail E. Nevin, P.T.
Janet A. Hulme, P.T.

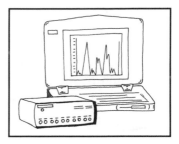

A biofeedback unit measures and displays information occurring within the body, information about body temperature (circulation to muscles), muscle tension (electrical activity of muscles), heart rate, and emotional response. This is information that a person doesn't normally perceive, information that is at an unconscious level. Biofeedback enables an individual to be aware of these processes at a conscious level. Circulation, muscle activity and breathing patterns are commonly altered in FMS, so with accurate information/feedback about these functions, the individual with FMS can learn the feeling of a normal activity level. Frequently returning to that normal level throughout the day can lead to a more pain-free, fatigue-free daily life. The person with FMS can gain back control over body functions that would otherwise limit quality of life, daily social interactions and vocational capabilities. Biofeedback gives fast, accurate audio or visual information about body signals normally ignored or not consciously perceived.

Blood Flow

In FMS, blood circulation to muscles of the back, arms, legs, hands and feet is often significantly decreased. Biofeedback gives accurate surface temperature information so FMS individuals can retrain blood vessels to dilate and increase blood flow to a body part.

Breathing

Feedback about minute by minute, hour by hour breathing is not typically at a conscious level, whether an individual has FMS or not. The diaphragm, the major breathing muscle, is often significantly affected in FMS and accessory muscles of the neck and upper chest and the intercostal muscles take over the breathing pattern. Electromyography (EMG) biofeedback gives accurate measurable information about diaphragmatic and accessory muscle activity during breathing. The FMS individual can reeducate the diaphragm and accessory muscles to restore normal function.

Muscle Activity

The resting level of an FMS individual's muscles in sitting, standing, or reclining position is generally high even though the brain's perception of the muscle resting level is that it is normal, quiet and relaxed. EMG biofeedback gives accurate, immediate sound or visual information to the conscious brain about muscle activity. Biofeedback supplements the internal message system with more accurate information about muscle activity at the conscious levels.

During daily activities such as cleaning, cooking, typing, even socializing the muscles used for these activities "overdo" or are at a higher level of activity than muscles of a non-FMS individual while accomplishing the same task. Surface EMG biofeedback gives information to the conscious brain centers so muscle activity can be modified via messages sent from the brain to the muscle fibers. The individual with FMS learns initially to check in using biofeedback equipment. Then later the biofeedback unit is replaced with use of internal sensation to assess muscles before, during, and after physical activities. That information is used to alter excessive activity, to learn "floating" techniques with the accurate information from external or internal biofeedback.

Stress Response

Biofeedback is also helpful in obtaining accurate information about and making changes in the response of the individual to stressors in daily life. The response of the FMS individual's heart, stomach, intestines, blood vessels, and sweat glands during daily stressors can be exaggerated or widely variable. The organs can be over or under active. Biofeedback is a tool that can be used to train the autonomic nervous system to stabilize these organs so function can be improved.

Sleep

Sleep disruption and fatigue are other major components of FMS. When there is a lack of restorative sleep in FMS the body is unable to repair and replace cell structures of all organ systems. Biofeedback is an important tool which assists the individual in consciously learning the patterns his/her body uses during rest and sleep, i.e., the muscle activity present, the breathing patterns used, and the circulation changes present. Biofeedback assists in training deep sleep.

Rest

Biofeedback is often essential for FMS individuals to use so they can learn what normal equilibrium is, what a normal physiological base line for muscles and internal organ functions is. Returning to that base line frequently throughout the day is the basis for a return to relatively pain-free, fatigue-free, daily life. Returning to that base line throughout the day means daily activities are accomplished with muscle and organ efficiency. With a return to resting base line soon after completion of any daily activity, energy can be conserved and utilized throughout the day instead of only for a short time. Efficiency and effectiveness of rest and sleep functions enable the individual to restore energy and capability for the following day.

For Clinicians Only

In the clinic situation biofeedback is used to improve the effectiveness and efficiency of assessing and treating individuals with FMS. Biofeedback is used to assess:

- muscle resting tone during:
  - sitting, standing and reclining
  - rest after completion of a muscle contraction
  - rest after completion of a functional activity
- muscle activity during:
  - rest
  - cognitive processing and mental stress
  - breathing
  - repeated muscle contraction
  - range of motion
  - functional activities
- circulation (hand temperature) during:
  - rest
  - a physical activity
  - rest after completion of 20-30 minutes of exercise

It is common to see muscle activity of FMS individuals compared to non FMS individuals:

- asymmetrical right vs left side at rest
- elevated at rest
- unable to return to rest after a physical activity or cognitive/emotional processing
- elevated during cognitive/emotional processing
- excessively elevated during physical activity
- inappropriate or excessive, i.e., cocontraction of muscles when inhibition is appropriate during physical activity
- inappropriate or excessive, i.e., use of associated muscles during physical activity that aren't necessary

It is common to see circulation of FMS individuals be:

- asymmetrical right vs left
- decreased at rest and during physical activity

The results of the assessment provide direction for re-education of muscle action and circulation. Treatment and self management goals based on the biofeedback assessment results include:

- improved muscle resting tone in sitting, standing, and reclining
- improved return to rest tone after exercise or functional activity
- improved symmetry of muscle resting tone
- improved muscle efficiency during functional activity or exercise
- improved muscle resting levels during cognitive and emotional processing
- improved symmetry of circulation right vs left
- improved circulation at rest and during physical exertion.

Clinical assessment and re education can be an effective part of an initial treatment protocol. Home biofeedback programs are just as essential to integrate the principles into daily life.

Chapter 10

What Can Psychotherapy Do To Help?

Ellen S. Silverglat, M.S.W.
Janet A. Hulme, P.T.

Counseling and/or psychotherapy can be of help in several areas including transitional issues, career/life planning, issues of lost function, spiritual direction and psychological testing. Counseling occurs in individual, couple, family, or group settings. Different types of counseling include cognitive-behavioral, regression therapy, hypnosis, and spiritual counseling.

Transitions

The person with FMS experiences numerous transitions accepting the condition and the changes it brings in self image, physical activity and time management. Living with a condition which is of indefinite duration is hard and until one can learn to think of time in more manageable quantities, it can be overwhelming. Talking with a person experienced in adjustment to chronic disease broadens the FMS individual's focus to include more than losses and negative change. Refocusing on positive aspects, what treatment can help and how to plan for both short and long term goals can diminish the feeling of hopelessness.

An illness that has no clear cut and predictable course really makes an individual feel out of control. In counseling, time is spent on rediscovering what you can do, how to make the "to do" list manageable, and what goals are realistic . . . all of which contribute to the feeling of regaining control and improved self esteem.

Counseling can help by addressing the global anxiety periodically experienced in FMS. The FMS individual may worry, "How can I make it through today? How will things be in the future?" Counseling teaches specific anxiety alleviating techniques that are very helpful in FMS.

Counseling assists in the treatment of depression that is common when there is significant long term pain. FMS individuals experience depression secondary to the chronic sleep disturbance, pain and fatigue. Some FMS individuals have a secondary diagnosis of clinical depression. In either case, the individual can be assisted by a psychotherapist and depression is treatable.

Types of Counseling

Psychological testing for memory problems and learning deficits can define the areas and extent of learning and processing problems and develop adaptations for school and work environments.

Counseling, especially cognitive-behavioral therapy, can help with accommodating changes in daily and weekly schedules. Cognitive-behavioral therapy teaches coping skills that help individuals control thoughts and actions that affect pain.

Regression therapy can assist the FMS individual in identifying early life events and family interactions that may be affecting how the person responds to daily life in the present.

Clinical hypnosis engages in a safe deep relaxation process, reaching a state of heightened awareness much like the edge of sleep, accessing the ability of the individual to reduce pain and fatigue.

Spiritual counseling involves pastoral assistance in the healing process.

Types of Counselors

A counselor, psychotherapist, psychiatrist or psychologist will assist in keeping things in perspective and help avoid seeing a catastrophe when a temporary setback is what has occurred.

Counseling is provided by certified or licensed mental health counselors, social workers, pastoral counselors, psychologists, and psychiatrists. In choosing a counselor it is important to interview the professional making sure they are educated about FMS, are compatible with the FMS individual, and interested in the same goals.

Group counseling can be very helpful and is often what occurs in support groups.

Support Groups

A support group can provide a sense of community for FMS individuals, a place to share the feelings, complaints, successes, treatments, and new research with others having the same chronic symptoms. A support group is also valuable for family members so they can gain information about the syndrome and begin to realize the encompassing symptoms as well as the variability and chronicity of FMS.

Newly diagnosed individuals can share feelings and questions with others who have experienced the fears and frustrations as well as the pain and fatigue. More experienced FMS individuals meet to share the latest management ideas, support each other in self care and provide emotional encouragement when there are exacerbations.

Support groups can organize calling circles or sponsors so anyone who needs it has a contact by phone when support is needed. Support groups often meet monthly for 1-2 hours utilizing part of the time for educational purposes and the rest for sharing between individuals.

Support groups, as they are active longer, can share information with the wider community through the print, radio, and TV media. They can also share with the health care community, government agencies and insurance companies through newsletters and workshops.

A new approach to support groups is through the computer internet. See Websites on page 230.

Chapter 11

What Tests Can I Do To Determine If My Body Systems Are In A Healthy State?

The basic assessment items the individual with fibromyalgia is asked to document are pain, stiffness and fatigue levels as indications of how they are doing. Additionally the individual may be asked to document the amount of exercise, housework or out of home work tolerated as indications of exercise tolerance. These are all components to look at in order to determine a healthy state. It is important to understand that these indicators are end products of physiological processes that precede the presence of FMS symptoms. The degree of dysfunction within the physiological processes correlates with the amount of pain, stiffness, and fatigue that an individual experiences.

Physiological Tests

Self tests that indicate the status of the underlying physiological processes include blood glucose levels, blood pressure and heart rate, breathing rate and pattern, muscle resting and work levels, basal body temperature, and menstrual cycle pattern. These parameters indicate how well the automatic control centers of the body are functioning to allow pain free, fatigue free work and daily activities. Rather than working until the pain or fatigue prevents function, it is now often possible to test certain physiological processes and make adjustments so pain and fatigue do not become the prevalent aspect of each day.

To treat fibromyalgia it is necessary to have testable signs that lead to appropriate intervention on a daily, sometimes even hourly basis. The goal is always to maintain that balance of the teeter-totter which then enables efficient body function for outside work and play.

Basic Self Tests	New Key indicator Self Tests
■ Pain Level	■ Blood Glucose Level
■ Fatigue Level	■ Basal Body Temperature
■ Sleep Patterns	■ Blood Pressure
■ Work Duration	■ Heart Rate
■ Tender Points	■ Breathing Pattern/Rate
	■ Muscle Resting Tone
	■ Menstrual Cycle Pattern
	■ Immune System Questionnaire

Combining the Basic Self Tests and the New Key Indicator Self Tests provides a compilation of data about the inner workings of each individual with FMS that is unprecedented. Using this information it is possible to respond more specifically and appropriately with interventions to prevent symptoms. When these tests are done on a frequent basis the interventions can occur before the teeter-totter becomes off balance and before the symptoms become limiting.

Baseline testing for 2-3 days can include all tests or only specific ones. Those tests that are indicative of imbalances for that individual are then placed in the Master Test Protocol (page 222). Each individual will have his/her own Master Test Protocol. For Mary, her Master Test Protocol included sleep patterns, muscle resting levels, and basal body temperature. For Bill the list included breathing rate, heart rate, and blood pressure. Both individuals also monitored pain and fatigue levels.

Pick 2-3 days that you are able to concentrate on your own needs. Then follow the Baseline Testing Procedure for Fibromyalgia.

82

Chapter 11: What Tests Can I Do To Determine
If My Body Systems Are In A Healthy State?

Baseline Testing Procedure for Fibromyalgia

First complete the General Fibromyalgia Criteria Questionnaire (see Chapter 2, page 21) including Associated Symptoms and Patterns and Variations. Summarize the results before proceeding to the Subcategory Questionnaire and Self Tests.

Key Indicator–Subcategory Assessment

Complete the Subcategory Characteristics Questionnaire. Then begin the Key Indicator Self Tests. Summarize the results on page 97.

Subcategory Characteristics Questionnaire

First fill in any boxes that describe your symptoms. Then circle one or two subcategories that most characterize you. If none are appropriate indicate that by circling General Symptoms Only.

Type 1a Hypoglycemia
☐ shakiness relieved by carbohydrates/sugar
☐ irritable/irrational
☐ craves sweets
☐ weakness

Type 1b Reactive Hypoglycemia
☐ shakiness relieved by protein/fat intake
☐ irritable/irrational
☐ craves fat/protein
☐ weakness

Type 2 Hypothyroid
☐ cold
☐ weight gain
☐ dry skin
☐ heavy periods
☐ hair loss
☐ constipation

Type 3 Neurally Mediated Hypotension
☐ dizzy
☐ low blood pressure
☐ increased heart rate/heart palpitations
☐ thirsty
☐ abdominal pain
☐ chest pain

Type 4 Immune System
☐ recurrent yeast infections
☐ frequent antibiotic use
☐ birth control pill use
☐ frequent cold sores
☐ frequent illnesses

Type 5 Reproductive Hormone
☐ monthly cycles of FMS pain & fatigue
☐ yearly cycles of FMS pain & fatigue
☐ PMS, menstrual pain/irregularity
☐ bowel & bladder irritability
☐ night sweats/hot flashes

Type G General Symptoms Only

Chapter 11: What Tests Can I Do To Determine
If My Body Systems Are In A Healthy State?

83

Key Indicator Tests of FMS Subcategories

Perform the Key Indicator Tests based on the Subcategory Types that you identified. For example, if Type 1 was your subcategory then use the Key Indicator Test for blood glucose levels to better identify the dysfunction. Perform each test for one to two days. If you have more than one subcategory you can do several tests at once or perform one test for a day or two and then another test for the next couple of days. The key indicator tests help to verify the subcategory. Once this has been completed, refer to page 89 to interpret your results.

1 Blood Glucose

Equipment: a blood glucose monitor. Follow the instructions on the unit. It can be purchased at a pharmacy.

Technique: Test your blood glucose level six times for 1-2 days and record results on the daily nutrition and glucose level chart.

- on awakening each morning
- prior to each meal
- 1 hour after each meal
- 3 hours after each meal if another meal has not been eaten
- prior to going to bed

It is very important that you record everything you eat and drink on the daily nutrition and glucose level chart and place the items on the hour when they are eaten. This enables a comparison of types of food eaten with glucose levels. Also, record how you feel mentally and physically at the time of each test.

2 Basal Body Temperature

Equipment: Oral thermometer.

Technique: In the morning before getting out of bed take your oral or underarm temperature. Before lunch and dinner and at bedtime record your oral or underarm temperature.

3 Heart Rate and Blood Pressure

Equipment: A heart rate and blood pressure monitor. Follow the instructions on the unit. It can be purchased at a pharmacy.

84

Chapter 11: What Tests Can I Do To Determine
If My Body Systems Are In A Healthy State?

Technique: Test your heart rate and blood pressure five times during the day. In the morning before you get out of bed, after breakfast, at lunch, at dinner, and before bedtime.

4 Immune System Questionnaire

Equipment: Immune System Questionnaire (page 87).

Technique: Answer the questions and record a summary of results. Is there indication of immune system dysfunction?

5 Menstrual Cycle Pattern (female only)

Equipment: Menstrual Cycle Questionnaire (page 87).

Technique: Summarize on the Daily Record Sheet the pattern of your menstrual cycle. Document how often you have a period, how long the period is, is it heavy or light, are there symptoms like pain or irritability related to the menstrual cycle? How many days before the cycle do they start? How long do they last? Do you experience yearly cycles of FMS symptoms i.e., worse during one part of the year, better during another?

6 Muscle Resting Tone

Equipment: Single channel or dual channel home surface electromyography (EMG) unit or Thermister. See Product Sources, page 229.

Technique: Three times a day record the (EMG) level of your neck/shoulder muscles. In the morning after breakfast sit in a comfortable chair, breathe naturally and record the EMG levels for 1-2 minutes. Then lift your shoulders toward your ears 5 times slowly and return to the rest position. Record how many seconds up to one minute it takes the muscles to return to the previous rest level after completing this activity. If the EMG does not return to the previous rest level within 1 minute record the rest level at the 1 minute time. In the afternoon after lunch record the EMG levels while standing up for 1-2 minutes. At night after dinner recline on your back and record the EMG levels for 1-2 minutes. Record the results on the EMG daily record sheet along with the pain and fatigue level at that time. This enables a comparison of muscle resting tone with pain and fatigue levels.

Chapter 11: What Tests Can I Do To Determine
If My Body Systems Are In A Healthy State?

85

At the present time EMG units are available by prescription only. If this is difficult to obtain the following test can be substituted. Hand temperature: use a Thermister to take your right and left hand temperature four times per day for 30-60 seconds each time. Take it before going to bed, before getting out of bed in the morning, and two other times during the day.

Breathing Pattern/Rate

Equipment: Watch with second hand, pen and paper.

Technique: Three times a day record your breathing pattern and rate for 1-2 minutes. For 15 seconds count the number of breaths and multiply by 4 to obtain the breaths per minute. Note where your breathing is occurring – in your abdomen, in your chest, in your neck and shoulders. Record all areas where you feel movement and breath on the daily breathing record sheet.

86

Chapter 11: What Tests Can I Do To Determine
If My Body Systems Are In A Healthy State?

◢4◣ Immune System Questionnaire

Check the box if answering yes to the question.

There is no definitive test used by medical physicians to determine immune system function. The diagnosis is most often based on history and symptoms. The questions from the medical history that are important include:

☐ Have you been treated with antibiotics especially for a month or longer or four or more times in a twelve month period?

☐ Have you experienced problems in your reproductive organs i.e., vaginitis, urethritis, prostatitis for more than a month?

☐ Have you ever had fungal infections such as athlete's foot, nail or skin fungal infection that lasted more than a month?

◢5◣ Menstrual Cycle Questionnaire

Check the box if answering yes to the question.

☐ Do you experience irregular periods? (Varies by more than 14 days from 28 days.)

☐ Do you experience periods longer than 7 days or shorter than 4 days? Which?_____

☐ Do you experience periods with either extremely heavy or very light menstrual flow? Which?_____

☐ Do you experience changes in pain, fatigue or irritability concurrent with your menstrual cycle?

☐ Do you experience changes in pain, fatigue or irritability concurrent with the seasons (fall/winter compared to spring/summer?)

Chapter 11: What Tests Can I Do To Determine
If My Body Systems Are In A Healthy State?

87

Daily Record Sheet

	1 Blood Pressure Rate	2 Blood Glucose Eaten	3 Basal Body Temp	Ⓖ Muscle Tone	Ⓖ Breathing Rate/ Location
Day 1					
Day 2					
Day 3					

Comments: _____

_____

_____

INTERPRETING THE TESTS

1 Blood Glucose Level

The glucose level in the blood is the sugar level in the blood that is available to interact with insulin and then be used by all cells of the body for energy. Normal blood glucose level is considered to be 80-120mg/dl. Clinical observation indicates optimal function for individuals with hypoglycemic or reactive hypoglycemic tendencies is 95 to 120 mg/dl. Optimal function of the body and mind occur between these levels. To maintain this level throughout the day insulin from the pancreas must be given off into the blood stream at a variable rate depending on many factors including the level of exercise, stress and the amount and type of food eaten. If too much insulin is given off it breaks down excessive blood sugar and the blood glucose level drops below the normal levels. This can be termed hypoglycemia or reactive hypoglycemia. If too little insulin is given off there remains too high a level of sugar in the blood stream since the small amount of insulin can combine with only a small portion of glucose. This is termed high blood glucose levels and can be indicative of diabetes. The symptoms of low blood sugar or hypoglycemia often include irritability, irrationality, physical fatigue, and muscle weakness. Additionally, as the reaction progresses sweating, increase in heart rate, dizziness and light-headedness, mental confusion, emotional outbursts, and extreme anxiety occur. Anger and resistance to others' suggestions is common. These symptoms are the result of low sugar (food) available to the brain, voluntary and autonomic nervous systems, and muscles.

Record the blood glucose levels in the daily record sheet using a glucometer and the blood from your knee or finger. Consult with your health care professional about the technique for using a glucometer.

Record the food you eat and the time you eat so a comparison can be made between the blood glucose reading and the type and amount of food you have taken in. During the days of record keeping engage in your normal physical exercise that is part of your daily routine. Be sure to indicate when and how much you exercise since this can affect blood glucose levels.

Chapter 11: What Tests Can I Do To Determine
If My Body Systems Are In A Healthy State?

89

Interpret Your Results

Looking at the data, ask yourself, "Is my blood glucose stable throughout the day or is there a large variation?" "Does my blood glucose level tend to be in the 80s or below, 80s and 90s, or 95 and above.?" "Does my blood glucose level ever go over 140?" "What do I feel like and what are the symptoms I am experiencing when my blood glucose test results are in the 80s or below? In the 90s, over 95?"

2 Basal Body Temperature

Basal body temperature is the heat created by the body's metabolism (fire). Normal basal body temperature is 98.6° F. If the body's metabolism is very low the body temperature will be decreased. If metabolism is high the body temperature will be increased. Heat is created within each cell of the body and is the result of the conversion of nutrients and chemicals into cellular energy. Even a small change in temperature affects cellular function significantly. Blood releases oxygen to the cells more readily at warmer temperatures and more slowly at cooler temperatures. Extreme temperature changes are life threatening. A decrease in body temperature to 97.6° F is significant enough to change physical and mental processes. The feeling of being cold, cold hands and feet, alternately feeling hot and cold, or sweating and shivering are common symptoms. Pain and mental confusion occur with longer term temperature decrease. More familiar are the symptoms associated with increased body temperature of which sweating, and feeling hot are the most common symptoms. Fatigue and lethargy occur with fever as well.

Interpret Your Results

Record your basal body temperatures on a predetermined basis. Ask these questions:

"Is my temperature lower or higher than the normal 98.6° F? If it is different is it consistently lower or higher or only at certain times of the day? How do I feel – cold, hot, energized, fatigued, painful, pain free?" Record a summary in the Interpretation Record.

90

Chapter 11: What Tests Can I Do To Determine
If My Body Systems Are In A Healthy State?

3 Blood Pressure/ Heart Rate

Blood pressure is the force of the blood traveling out of the heart and down the arteries of the body. Normal blood pressure for adults less than 60 years old is 150/90mm/hg. Consistent readings above 150/90mm/hg are considered high blood pressure. Consistent readings below 100/70mm/hg is considered low blood pressure. 120mm/hg is the pressure of the ventricle pushing the blood into the ascending aorta, 80mm/hg is the pressure in the blood vessel in between beats. Heart rate at rest averages 60-70 beats per minute (bpm) on the average. Resting heart rate above 90 beats per minute is considered excessive. Blood pressure and heart rate are controlled to a large extent by the autonomic nervous system. Record your blood pressure and heart rate in the daily record sheet.

Interpret Your Results

Answer the questions, " Is my heart rate above 90 bpm at rest? Is my blood pressure normal, high or low? Does my blood pressure and/or heart rate change with different positions? Does my blood pressure or heart rate vary greatly or remain stable?" Record your comments in the Interpretation Report including any symptoms you or those around you perceive as occurring when you take your blood pressure and heart rate.

4 Immune System Dysfunction

The immune system helps to control the body's health and wellness. The indication of repeated or excessive use of antibiotics, repeated infections or illnesses, repeated or chronic emotional stressors, chemical or environmental stressors can significantly impact the immune system function. The immune system responds to stressors with increased activation but eventually fatigues and "shuts down" or depresses in function if adequate rest is not available.

Interpret Your Results

Record in the Interpretation Record a summary of the questions you answered a 'yes' to from the Immune System Questionnaire on page 87.

Chapter 11: What Tests Can I Do To Determine
If My Body Systems Are In A Healthy State?

91

5 Menstrual Cycle Pattern

The menstrual cycle is a cyclical hormonal change usually over a 28-30 day period in females. The hormones given off by the reproductive organs during the menstrual cycle affect all body systems. During the menstrual cycle estrogen and progesterone vary through a 28 day period. During the first 14 days estrogen is produced at a higher level than progesterone stimulating a rise in blood level carbon dioxide from the onset of menstruation to ovulation. During the second 14 days progesterone is produced at a higher level than estrogen resulting in decreased blood levels of carbon dioxide until menstruation begins again. A rise in progesterone during the last 14 days increases basal body temperature and respiratory rate. In addition to the monthly hormonal cycle in women there is a yearly cycle. In the spring there is a general rise in estrogen production and during the late fall there is a decline in estrogen production. When there is a disruption in the hormonal cycle, (the ratio of estrogen to progesterone changes or there is a chronically low level of both hormones) the effect on body temperature, breathing rate, muscle function, brain function, and intestinal activity can be significant since these hormones affect all cellular function.

Interpret Your Results

Record on the Interpretation Record a summary of the questions you answered 'yes' to from the Menstrual Cycle Questionnaire (page 87). Ask yourself the following questions, "Do I have regular menstrual cycles? If there are irregularities what are they? Are my fibromyalgia symptoms increased or decreased in relation to my menstrual cycle? How?"

G Breathing Pattern/Rate

An individual's breathing is automatic and the pattern and rate are generally similar for everyone. At rest 10-12 breaths per minute is within normal limits. Breathing is designed to provide oxygen for use by the body cells in burning fuels for energy and function. It is designed to excrete waste products like carbon dioxide. Oxygen and carbon dioxide are essential for function but are toxic when present in excess. The acidity of the body is largely determined by the level of carbon dioxide in the blood stream. Virtually all metabolic processes depend on adequate acid-base balance. Increased carbon dioxide is correlated with nervous system hyperexcitability – muscles are hyperirritable, pupils dilate, extremities are cold, and there is increased sweating. During hyperventilation (shallow breathing with loss of carbon dioxide) blood flow to the brain, hands, feet, and intestines decreases. This can affect thinking and memory, digestion and absorption of food as well as coordination and ambulation. Hyperventilation has been linked to a sudden dramatic decrease in blood pressure which may result in syncope or fainting. Breathing also affects heart rate and cellular metabolism. Breathing is automatic, you do not have to think about each breath. If you had to think about each breath it would be hard to get anything else done during the day. During exercise your breathing rate increases and during meditation or sleep it decreases. Diaphragmatic breathing is the most efficient form of breathing. During diaphragmatic breathing, as you inhale your diaphragm descends and the abdomen will rise or move outward. As you exhale the diaphragm will return to the dome shape and the abdomen will move inward. The diaphragm is descending into the abdominal cavity with inhalation and ascending or rising towards the breastbone with exhale. During diaphragmatic breathing the upper chest and shoulders are quiet and the abdominal muscles are relatively relaxed. The jaw is released, the teeth separated, and the tongue is relaxed at the bottom of the mouth, the tip of the tongue resting lightly behind the top front teeth. Hyperventilation is characterized by rapid chest breathing. Irregular breathing cycles, sighing, and interrupted breathing (apnea) can also occur.

Interpret Your Results

Record the interpretation of your typical breathing noticing where the breathing occurs – in the neck, shoulders, chest, abdomen or diaphragm. If you noticed movement in your upper chest and/or shoulders during breathing the accessory muscles of neck and chest are being used for each breath. Then record the pattern of your breathing. Normal breathing pattern is equal inhale and exhale with slight rest between each. Ask yourself, "Do I inhale and exhale equally or is my inhale longer or shorter than my exhale?" "Do I yawn a lot? Do I feel out of breath at rest or doing quiet activities?" Yawning and shortness of breath may indicate an abnormal breathing pattern.

Chapter 11: What Tests Can I Do To Determine
If My Body Systems Are In A Healthy State?

93

Is your breathing rate average, slower or faster than the average? Do you breathe using the breathing diaphragm or using the neck, chest and shoulder muscles? What is your breathing pattern – the inhale to exhale ratio? Record your interpretation of breathing pattern, rate, and location on the Interpretation Record.

G Muscle Resting Tone

The muscle resting level is the tension or tone in the muscles when they are at rest and not doing a physical activity. Even at rest each muscle holds some tone but for efficient healthy body function this resting tone needs to be consistently low and slow. In other words the muscle tone is relaxed and the readiness to respond is present but not excessively vigilant. The first area to assess is the resting level of the muscles in different positions. Using the results from the home bio-feedback unit, notice if the EMG levels are the same or different as you change positions from sitting to standing to reclining. Then notice if they were different from day to day. A difference is expected when you change position because gravity pulls on muscles and the muscles respond by "pulling back". Therefore standing usually exhibits the highest muscle resting tone and reclining exhibits the lowest. Daily variations should be small since an individual with a balanced body system rests effectively at relatively the same level unless there is a major stressor on a particular day.

The next area to assess is how quickly and effectively the muscles return to the resting level after working during an activity. After raising and lowering your shoulders 5 times how many seconds did it take for the shoulder/neck muscles to return to the previous rest level? Efficient, effective muscles can return to rest within seconds and remain in the rest level until another activity is required. If a muscle takes more than 10-20 seconds to return to rest or is erratic in being able to maintain the rest level unnecessary energy is used and the elevated tone can lead to pain and fatigue.

The temperature of fingers and hands is determined by the amount of blood flowing into the area. If the blood vessels are open and dilated, hands are warm. If the blood vessels are closed and restricted, hands are cooler. The blood vessel walls are lined with muscle so when the resting tone is high the walls are constricted and the hands will be

94

Chapter 11: What Tests Can I Do To Determine
If My Body Systems Are In A Healthy State?

cooler. When the muscle resting tone is low the hands will be warm. The tone in arm, leg and back muscles usually correlates with muscle tone in the blood vessels, therefore, hand temperature will most often correlate with muscle tone. One side of the body may have a different temperature than the other. One side of the body may have more muscle tone than the other. Temperature may vary through the day and night. Normal hand temperature is 94 to 96° F.

Interpret Your Results

Record your interpretation of muscle resting level in sitting, standing and reclining on the Interpretation Report. Also record your interpretation of return to rest after an activity. Record your interpretation of hand temperatures. Is your right and left hand the same or different? Does your hand temperature vary throughout the day? Do you notice your hands feeling cold?

Chapter 11: What Tests Can I Do To Determine
If My Body Systems Are In A Healthy State?

95

INTERPRETATION RECORD

☐1 **BLOOD GLUCOSE LEVEL**

☐2 **BASAL BODY TEMPERATURE**

☐3 **BLOOD PRESSURE/HEART RATE**

☐4 **IMMUNE SYSTEM QUESTIONNAIRE**

☐5 **MENSTRUAL CYCLE**

☐6 **BREATHING PATTERN/RATE**

☐7 **MUSCLE RESTING LEVEL**

Now it is possible to identify which tests indicated changes in your body function that relate to physical and mental symptoms labeled fibromyalgia symptoms. List the Key Indicator Tests that demonstrate changes from normal levels. Identify the subcategory(ies) that are closest to your characteristics using the Key Indicators and the Subcategory Questionnaire.

My Key Indicators are:

1.
2.
3.

My Subcategory(ies) are:

1.
2.

With this knowledge it is possible to minimize the fibromyalgia symptoms by normalizing the body functions that are presently abnormal. For example, if Type 2 Hypothyroid Tendency is the characteristic subcategory and basal body temperature is low and variable then techniques to stabilize and increase the basal body temperature can often significantly decrease the fibromyalgia symptoms. If Type 1 Hypoglycemia Tendency is the characteristic sub-category and blood glucose levels are low then methods to stabilize and increase blood glucose levels can significantly decrease the fibromyalgia symptoms. There may be one or more Key Indicators that you decide are important to monitor. These Key Indicators will be the ones you continue to test as you progress through the self care treatment phase of this protocol.

The Next Step

The next step in the process is to combine your major characteristics and associated symptoms with your key indicators and subcategories on the Personal Profile Summary (page 99). Once you have completed the Personal Profile Summary go to Chapter 12 and proceed with the Self Care Stabilizing Loop for General Fibromyalgia. Each succeeding chapter describes in detail the subcategory type and the Self Stabilizing Loop that benefits that group of individuals with FMS. Take it step by step. As the General Fibromyalgia Self Care Stabilizing Loop becomes easy, proceed to the Subcategory Chapter(s). Retest the key indicators of that subcategory and begin that Self Care Stabilizing Loop, adding it to the General Self Care you are already doing.

Chapter 11: What Tests Can I Do To Determine
If My Body Systems Are In A Healthy State?

97

The FMS Treatment Flow Chart leads you step by step through the progression of activities.

FMS Self Care Flow Chart

Check off each item as you complete it. There is no hurry to go to the next step. Take your time and get to know your special needs.

☐   Identify items on the Fibromyalgia Criteria Check List that are characteristic of your symptoms (Chapter 2, page 21)

☐   Identify your Key Indicators (page 97)

☐   Identify your Subcategory(ies) (page 97)

☐   Begin Basic Self Stabilizing Loop self care techniques (Chapter 12)

☐   Assess benefits and make changes as needed

☐   Begin Subcategory Self Stabilizing Loop(s) self care techniques and monitor your Key Indicator(s) (Chapter 13)

☐   Assess benefits and make changes as needed

☐   Develop your individualized Self Stabilizing Loop (Chapter 15-19). Record your tests and protocol on page 222.

Once you have summarized your characteristics and determined possible subcategory(ies) you may then read the appropriate chapters and begin the sequence of self care techniques that can help your symptoms. Begin with one or two techniques and repeat those until they are fairly easy before adding new ones. It is important to assess which techniques help and continue to use those. Self care techniques that are not effective are dropped or altered.

98

Chapter 11: What Tests Can I Do To Determine
If My Body Systems Are In A Healthy State?

PERSONAL PROFILE SUMMARY

MY MAJOR CHARACTERISTICS
& ASSOCIATED SYMPTOMS

1. _____
   _____
   _____

2. _____
   _____
   _____

3. _____
   _____
   _____

4. _____
   _____
   _____

5. _____
   _____
   _____

MY KEY INDICATORS:

1. _____
   _____

2. _____
   _____

3. _____
   _____

MY SUBCATEGORIES:

1. _____
   _____
   _____

2. _____
   _____
   _____

Chapter 12

▨ What Can I Do To Manage Fibromyalgia Through Self Care

Joyce Dougan, P.T.
Barbara Penner, P.T.
Gail E. Nevin, P.T.
Janet A. Hulme, P.T.

Self Stabilizing Loops

The knowledge available from your Personal Profile (page 99) enables you to begin managing your FMS more effectively. The goal of any individual with fibromyalgia symptoms is to function well and fully in daily life, in work, social, recreational, and family activities with pain-free energy. This goal, at the physiological level, requires efficient and effective muscle work and rest cycles. Muscles of the arms, legs, back, abdomen and neck – the voluntary muscles – must function efficiently and effectively. Additionally, smooth muscles of the heart, lungs, gut, bladder and reproductive organs that are controlled by the autonomic nervous system must function efficiently to accomplish pain-free daily activities. To optimize the function of muscles it is necessary for them to receive and absorb the essential nutrients and oxygen needed for energy production (metabolism) within their cell structures and to effectively eliminate the waste products left after the metabolic process is completed. The goal is to achieve normal function in daily and work activities, in leisure time activities, and during sleep.

Treatment

Ideally you are working with a health care professional to set your goals and monitor progress of each treatment approach. It is important to find a trusted and interested professional to be your coach and guide you in your recovery. Treatment can include medication and self care. No pill, surgery, or counseling has proven to be a cure. Medications can help but in most cases medication does not completely alleviate the symptoms over the long term. Self care becomes the primary treatment to alleviate the symptoms of fibromyalgia and optimize functional and work activities.

It is common for an individual with fibromyalgia to comment, "I am too busy with my family and work to do all that self care stuff," or "I did the self care routine for several months and got better but it didn't last when I went back to my usual routine," or "My family (spouse) thinks I am being selfish and self centered when I spend so much time on me." With these comments it is no wonder that the best treatment is often ignored.

Self care is a form of work, a job that must come first if the individual is to function optimally in the home, family and work place. It is a job that must be maintained over the life time. The individual brushes her teeth and washes her face every day as a given part of life. The self care routine for fibromyalgia is the same as brushing and washing. It is forever and important. The individual with fibromyalgia deserves to include those self care items that provide health and enable her/him to function in a healthy way with family and society.

Sometimes the individual is able to gradually integrate the self care routine into life activities without changing the daily routine much. Other times it is necessary to interrupt the normal routine for a time and emphasize self care to realize what being a healthy person can feel like. Then family, social and work activities are gradually added back in when the self care routine is effectively in place. It is important that the self care routine remain at the core of daily life. It is not an add on when there is time.

Case Study

Mary tells of using self care techniques in a concentrated way for six weeks and feeling a lot better, sleeping, exercising, using Physiological Quieting, changing her nutritional patterns. Then her physician told her she could go back to work. Her family said they were glad she was well now and could start doing what she did before. Her coworkers welcomed her back and she returned to her same job. Within two weeks she was exhausted, aching and painful and expressed confusion and frustration about what to do now.

The answer to the scenario described above is continual self care.

Self care is the best solution to a chronic problem. It needs to be a deserved priority on a daily basis. There will still be ups and downs but the windows of "feeling good" will be larger and the crisis times will be less intense.

To discover the best self care approach for each individual takes time and exploration. Each individual will be unique in his/her needs in spite of similarities throughout the population as a whole.

When a new technique like exercise is started, it is important to start slowly and gradually increase the intensity and repetitions. As with any other sensory input, the fibromyalgia nervous system over-responds to the sensation and action of new events. That can exhaust the body and mind quickly or set off the teeter-totter imbalance within the many body systems. Floating through exercises, doing a few repetitions of each exercise, and emphasizing rest as much as work is the basic rule for all new endeavors. Work and recreational related activities must be approached the same way. Constantly quieting the systems keeps the balance and prevents increased pain, fatigue and dysfunction.

To get started on your program of healthy living remember you were made a deserving human being and your most important job is to care for your body and mind in the ways it needs to be healthy. There cannot be a separation between the body and mind, the body is equal to the mind in value, intelligence and work capabilities and deservedness.

⚡ The General FMS Self Stabilizing Loop

The Basic Self Stabilizing Loop includes the self care spiral
(Figure 9)

- Sleep Routine
- Physiological Quieting
- Nutrition
- Exercise
- Medication
- Positive Self Talk

- Rest/Work Cycles
- Pacing/Prioritizing
- Dress
- Modalities
- Journaling

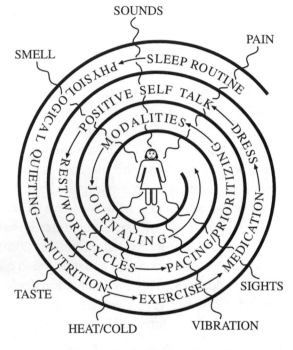

Figure 9: Self Care Spiral

The General Fibromyalgia Self Care Stabilizing Loop items are listed in priority order. Sleep protocol, Physiological Quieting, and Nutrition are combined in the first step. It may take several weeks to a month to develop these new behaviors. No one can expect to turn over a new leaf in a day or a week. Persevering along a path of small steps and positive actions will result in decreased symptoms. Check off the items as you progress through the First Step Protocol on page 105.

🄶 General FMS Self Care Stabilizing Loop

	M	T	W	T	F	S	S	Comments
First Step Protocol								
<u>Sleep</u>								
Defined bedtime/rise time								
8-9 hours/sleep								
snack at bedtime								
remove caffeine								
PQ at bedtime								
appropriate bed clothing and pillows								
environmental stimuli stabilized								
<u>Physiological Quieting</u>								
listen to PQ tape at night								
hourly PQ for 30 seconds								
<u>Nutrition</u>								
reduce/eliminate simple sugars								
caffeine								
alcohol								
6-8 glasses water daily								
vitamin / mineral food / supplements								
amino acid foods/supplements								
reduce/eliminate detrimental foods								
Second Step Protocol								
<u>Exercise</u>								
20-30 min. daily								
<u>Medication</u>								
1.								
2.								
3.								
<u>Positive Self Talk</u>								
1.								
2.								
3.								
<u>Rest/Work Cycles</u>								
<u>Pacing/Prioritize</u>								
<u>Dress</u>								
<u>Modalities</u>								
<u>Journaling</u>								

Sleep Protocol

Sleep is the most important first step in health for individuals with fibromyalgia. Deep sleep occurs when there is replacement and repair of all cells of body and mind. During sleep it is important that your body systems remain relatively stable. For example:

- your temperature needs to remain relatively stable,
- your blood sugar needs to remain relatively stable,
- your muscle tension/tightness needs to remain relatively relaxed,
- your mind activity needs to remain relatively quiet,
- your oxygen levels need to remain relatively stable.

To that end self care techniques that help these systems remain stable will be the first ones to learn and integrate into daily life. These include:

- Physiological Quieting (PQ) – breathing, hand warming, and PQ audiotape (page 108)
- Eliminate nutritional stimulants – caffeine, alcohol
- Minimize environmental irritants – noise, odor, temperature, light
- Schedule regular and adequate time for sleep.

As these become regular habits in daily life, pain, fatigue, and associated symptoms can significantly decrease.

Since restful sleep is a top priority for FMS individuals, planning an individual routine for sleep is important. "I want to be able to get to sleep, sleep through the night without pain and frequent waking. I want to feel rested and limber when I awake," Jody tells her health care consultant.

To get to sleep:

- Remove stimulants such as caffeine from your diet. This includes any coffee, tea, soda or chocolate that contains caffeine. Some headache and pain remedies contain caffeine and should be changed to another non-caffeine containing medication. Caffeine is a stimulant to the autonomic nervous system, increasing pain perception, stimulating the brain's arousal systems and facilitating wakefulness. It is also a bladder irritant so it can increase the times you need to go to the bathroom at night.
- Hunger and/or hypoglycemia can increase insomnia symptoms so eating a light carbohydrate snack like a piece of whole wheat toast

or a banana along with a small amount of a milk product or protein just before bedtime can improve sleep. Milk products contain tryptophan, a natural chemical that has a calming and relaxing affect on the nervous system and is a precursor to serotonin. Milk products also contain calcium which helps with sleep and muscle relaxation. Carbohydrates help speed tryptophan to the brain.

- A regular bedtime and wake up time is important for individuals with sleep disturbance. Eight to ten hours of sleep each night is important. Growth hormone in FMS individuals is produced in greatest amounts during the early morning hours, so the best sleep for FMS is sometimes termed "sleeping in" by others. Growth hormone is essential for the growth and repair of all body cells. Shift changes at a job are not conducive to health with FMS individuals since the body clock needs to practice the same routine over a long period of time and is hypersensitive to disruption.

- The hour before bedtime needs to be a time of winding down, a time for yourself and quiet enjoyment. It is not a time to be balancing the checkbook, paying the bills, or settling a family disagreement. Instead, try soft music, a hot bath, a good book, or writing in a journal. This is the time to use Physiological Quieting in preparation for sleep.

To stay asleep:

- Use a supportive mattress that has its own soft pad or place an egg crate mattress under the sheet and mattress pad. Try different pillows until you find the best one for your head and neck, one that is most comfortable through the night and enables you to wake up with minimal feelings of stiffness and soreness in your neck and shoulders. Use a pillow between your knees and hug one when you sleep on your side. When sleeping on your back, place pillows under your knees as well as supporting your head and neck. You may even want pillows to support each shoulder and arm. Sleeping on your stomach is not recommended because of the extreme position it puts your neck and low back.

- Wear warm night wear with long sleeves and long pants. Some people even wear socks, gloves and nightcaps to help maintain body temperature while sleeping.

- Warm the bed before you get in using a heating pad or electric mattress pad. Turn it off before you go to sleep.
- Eliminate environmental factors that can arouse a light sleeper. Dark out shades and a sleep mask keep out light. A sound conditioner which produces white noise or ear plugs block out the background noise of car engines, horns, and people talking. Essential oils such as lavendar and eucalyptus can facilitate restfulness and block out other stimulating smells. Stabilize the room heat so the temperature is the same all night and use blankets which are adequate for the duration of sleep.
- Exercise moderately 20-30 minutes some time during the day at least three hours before bedtime. Exercising in the evening stimulates the nervous system and may increase alertness and wakefulness.
- If you wake up during the night move to a comfortable position, then relax muscles head to toe into the bed and begin diaphragmatic breathing, hand warming, and positive self statements. Know that your body and mind are in a restful state even if you do not perceive that you are asleep.
- If you can't get back to sleep after a half an hour to an hour get up, read a book, write in a journal, or do some gentle exercise, and then try to sleep again later.
- Use prescribed medication consistently. Consult a physician about changes in sleep patterns.

The goal: **sleep through the night, wake rested and limber!**

Physiological Quieting

An individual responds to events in daily life through chemical changes within the body and brain. The alarm in the morning is perceived by the ear, transferred to the brain center for hearing by chemical events within the nerve, then interpreted by the head and gut control centers which send messages to the rest of the body through additional chemicals saying, "open your eyes, jump out of bed, get dressed." Chemical messages are different depending on how the event is perceived by the head and gut brain. If the event is perceived as an emergency, a fight or flight event, chemicals such as adrenaline and testosterone are released in increased amounts; if the event is perceived as a normal, easy life event by the brain and body the chemicals released are different and give activating but calmer directions to all organs and tissues.

FMS individuals' brain centers and nervous systems tend to respond to life events with excessive fight or flight chemicals rather than quieting chemicals. The autonomic nervous system that controls heart rate, breathing, stomach and intestine activity, bladder function, and circulation tends to send out more fight or flight chemicals than quieting chemicals. We say it has a high idle at rest, always ready to jump. The on/off switch for full activation is hypersensitive. This means even normal daily events may activate chemical messengers that are meant for use only during short periods of high stress. This constant activation of stress chemicals is destructive to the body over the long term. Circulation to muscles is decreased so muscles ache from lack of oxygen and accumulation of waste products. Breathing rate increases and breathing is shallow and irregular so the FMS individual complains of shortness of breath and low endurance during aerobic activity. Heart rate increases and is often irregular, chest pain and pressure are experienced. Stomach and intestinal activity increases. Excessive abnormal smooth muscle contractions can cause stomach and abdominal pain, diarrhea, and indigestion. Light, irregular sleep can prevent repair and replacement of body cells.

It is important to use management techniques that quiet the high idle or high resting level of the nervous system. It is important to use management techniques that assist the autonomic nervous system in responding to daily events with "calm" chemical messengers to organ systems instead of "fight or flight" chemical messengers.

These techniques are termed Physiological Quieting. Physiological Quieting (PQ) is an integral part of a successful FMS management system. Its goals are:

- to rebalance the autonomic nervous system regulation of circulation and internal organ function (heart, lungs, intestines),
- to normalize the release of chemical messengers from the head and gut control centers to the rest of the body, and
- to equalize the feedback message loop from the body to the head compared to the message loop from the head to the body telling it what to do, what it needs for health and well being.

The divisions of the autonomic nervous system (ANS) are the sympathetic, the parasympathetic, and the enteric (gut). The ANS directs/regulates the activity of all organs of the body. When this "body-brain" feedback loop is balanced, the individual is in a state of health. When the body-brain feedback loop is unbalanced, the individual is in a state of dis-ease. It is important to balance the body messages with the head messages, to balance the sympathetic (fight or flight) messages with the parasympathetic (quieting) messages, and the gut (enteric) messages with the head (CNS) messages to have optimal health for FMS individuals. An overactive sympathetic nervous system leads to decreased circulation, increased muscle resting tone (both smooth and striated), and myofascial tissue thickening (Figure 10) which results in pain, fatigue, and limitations of daily activities.

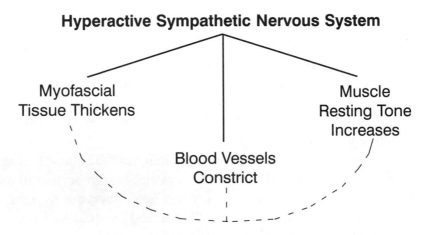

Figure 10: Hyperactive Sympathetic Nervous System

With a well balanced autonomic nervous system and with smooth running feedback loops between body and brain, sleep improves, muscle function improves, circulation improves, and pain and fatigue diminish. Physiological Quieting techniques are targeted to balance the autonomic nervous system and its feedback loops with the central nervous system. The three major techniques in Physiological Quieting are:

- Breathing
- Hand Warming
- Body/Mind Quieting

Breathing

Approximately ten to fifteen percent of FMS individuals have a sense of dyspnea (air hunger) even in a resting state. During exercise an FMS individual's breathing pattern is irregular when normal individuals would have extremely regular breathing. The diaphragm, the major breathing muscle, becomes dysfunctional much as other muscles do in FMS. Accessory breathing muscles in the neck and chest take over for the diaphragm. Breathing affects tissue oxygen levels, body metabolism, heart rate and the body's acid base balance. When breathing is erratic and the muscle action producing breathing patterns is changed, these physiological processes are severely altered. Heart rate is increased, nerve/muscle resting level is elevated, and blood pressure changes due to breathing changes. Symptoms described by FMS individuals that can be directly attributed to hyperventilation, the most drastic form of erratic breathing, include: shortness of breath, chest pain, choking or smothering sensation, dizziness, numbness and tingling in hands and feet, hot and cold flashes, faintness, trembling, and fear or anxiety feelings. With this in mind, returning to diaphragmatic breathing becomes an important aspect of FMS management.

Basic Exercise

The diaphragm is a large sheetlike muscle that rests in a dome shape in the chest from the nipple area to the bottom of the rib cage and the spine. As you inhale the dome flattens and pulls down to the bottom of the rib cage. During exhale the diaphragm moves back to the dome shape. When breathing correctly, the shoulder and chest areas remain quiet, the jaw is relaxed, and the teeth are separated. Inhale, 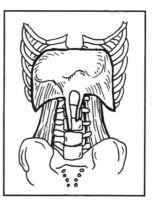 let your abdomen rise, exhale, let it fall. There is equal time for inhale and exhale. Inhaling through the nose, exhaling through the mouth or nose. Exhale is passive and quiet.

Diaphragmatic breathing eases and reverses the biochemical effects of hyperventilation and makes it easier for air to flow into the lungs. Practice diaphragmatic breathing initially in a reclined position, then in sitting and standing. Practice hourly during the day, 7-8 breaths.

Advanced Exercise

An advanced breathing exercise that helps to normalize diaphragm muscle function in relation to other body functions is the following:

- In a comfortable, supported position focus on low, slow diaphragmatic breathing.
- Now add: arch low back slightly with inhale, flatten low back with exhale.
- When this is easy add: roll legs out slightly with inhale, roll legs in with exhale.
- When this is easy add: roll palms up with inhale, roll palms down with exhale.
- When this is easy add: rock chin up slightly with inhale, rock chin down with exhale.

Practice 5-10 of these total body breaths in the morning before you get up and as you go to sleep at night.

Hand Warming

Circulation to muscles, nerves, internal organs, and the brain is often significantly decreased in FMS individuals. Some FMS individuals describe being core cold, not being able to warm up. Their hands and feet are cold, their buttocks feel cold, even their internal organs feel cold. Often a cold feeling is a cardinal sign of worsening FMS symptoms of muscle aching and fatigue within the next 6-8 hours.

Decreased circulation means blood vessel constriction. Blood vessel walls have three layers, one of which is muscular. The muscular layer is controlled by the sympathetic (fight or flight) nervous system. An active sympathetic system causes constriction of the blood vessel wall, a quieting sympathetic system causes dilation or relaxation of the blood vessel wall, allowing more blood flow. When more blood flows through the vessels there is increased heat from the increased blood volume which results in hands, feet and other body parts warming. This increases circulation to all muscles, bringing in food and oxygen and carrying away waste products so muscles can function with greater energy and less pain and fatigue.

Hand warming is a technique to increase blood volume to body parts. Mental imaging and frequently repeated thoughts transfer to nerve activity that quiets the sympathetic (fight or flight) nervous system activity resulting in dilation of blood vessels. To accomplish this:

- Visualize the warmest place your hands can be, holding a warm cup of hot chocolate, holding your hands over a camp fire or radiator, or slipping your hands and feet in the hot sand of a beach on a summer day.
- Think of the warmest color and surround your hands and wrists with that color. Let that color flow into your hands, deep into the palms, fingers, wrists while they get warmer and warmer.
- Focus your attention on your hands and say to yourself, "My hands are warmer and warmer, warmth is flowing into my hands, warmer and warmer."

To accomplish a resetting of the autonomic nervous system, to slow the high idle, it is necessary to practice the techniques that quiet the sympathetic system frequently for short periods. The instructions are:

"Practice hourly for 30-60 seconds, wherever you are. No one will know you are doing it." Put colored dots up around your work and home or buy a watch that buzzes every hour to remind you. Then hourly do:

- 7-8 slow, low diaphragmatic breaths
- Release jaw, quiet shoulders quiet chest
- 7-8 repetitions of hand warming

Body/Mind Quieting

Balancing the ANS (body control centers) with the CNS (head control centers) helps all organs and muscles be their healthiest. The head is used to bossing the body around. It is not used to listening to what the body needs and has to say. Initially it will take conscious practice to re-connect the body to mind message system.

However, with practice it will become automatic for the feedback loop between the body to the head to be as strong as the head to the body (Figure 11).

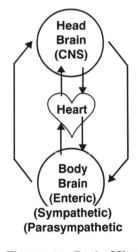

Figure 11: Body-Mind Feedback Loop

Body/mind quieting serves many important functions in helping FMS individuals. Excessive muscle resting levels and internal organ activity can be decreased through Physiological Quieting of the body/mind. Abnormal sleep patterns are improved with Physiological Quieting of the body/mind. Physiological Quieting of the body/mind assists the immune system in optimal functioning.

To accomplish body/mind quieting:

Find a quiet, warm room with a chair or bed that gives complete support from your head to your feet. Use pillows for support of your neck, low back, arms, and knees.

- Focus on your breathing, feel the pattern of breathing, let your abdomen rise with inhale, fall with exhale.
- Feel the warmth or coolness of your hands and feet, left side and right. Let your hands and feet feel warm, feel warmer and warmer.
- Feel the support of the bed or chair and release into that support, let your feet, legs, hips, back, shoulders, arms, neck and head sink deeper and deeper into that support.
- Focus on your face and neck. Notice where there is any tension or tightness, where there is quiet, calmness in each part of your face and neck muscles - your forehead, eyes, cheeks, tongue, throat, neck. Then say to yourself 3-4 times slowly, "My face and neck muscles are quiet and calm, my face and neck muscles are calmer and calmer."
- Proceed from head to toe in the same manner, focusing on head and neck, back (upper, middle and lower), shoulders and arms, hips and legs, chest and abdomen.
- Focus again on diaphragmatic breathing and hand warming.

One to two 20 minute body/mind quieting sessions a day are recommended. Try doing it 20 minutes before you get out of bed in the morning and 20 minutes before going to sleep at night using the Physiological Quieting audiotape.

Integrating Physiological Quieting throughout the day is an essential aspect of self care in FMS management.

Nutrition

The nutritional component in managing FMS can be controversial. Mary is told by her dietician to "eat a normal diet based on the food group pyramid." Jolene consults several traditional and alternative health care providers and uses nutritional supplements in addition to a balanced diet. The goal of good nutrition in FMS is to provide the needed food products that can be broken down and utilized for optimal body functions.

Nutrition is the next step in health for individuals with fibromyalgia. It comes before exercise because without adequate nutrition the muscle cells cannot function to perform exercise. The nutrients taken in through food and supplements are broken down and converted to usable substances by the digestive system. Considerations in healthy body use of nutritional components includes:

- adequate intake of needed nutrients
- elimination of detrimental nutrients
- adequate digestion of needed nutrients
- adequate absorption of needed nutrients
- adequate transportation of needed nutrients to body/ mind cells
- adequate metabolism of nutrients by cells for optimal cellular function

Adequate intake of needed nutrients can be different for each individual. There are general guidelines to begin with but it is trial and error to find out what works best for each individual's systems. General guidelines include:

- intake of water 6-8 glasses daily, 1 glass every 30 minutes of exercise
- regularly scheduled meals with balanced nutrient intake
- adequate vitamins, minerals, essential fatty acids, essential amino acids

Elimination of detrimental nutrients include:

- minimize caffeine – coffee, tea, chocolate, caffeinated soda
- minimize alcohol
- minimize sugar intake

Adequate digestion of needed nutrients is determined by the digestive system from the mouth to the rectum and anus. Considerations include:

- chewing ability in the mouth
- swallowing ability
- stomach digestion – breakdown of fruits
- small intestine digestion – breakdown of fats, carbohydrates
- colon function – absorption of water and nutrients
- rectum and anus – elimination of waste products

Individuals with fibromyalgia often complain of jaw/tooth pain which can change chewing habits. Chewing is the first step in digestion. Swallowing difficulties are common complaints in fibromyalgia. Choking and pain with swallowing affects what foods are eaten. Chest pain, stomach pain, and burping can be symptoms of stomach digestive problems. When stomach and small intestine digestion is affected, absorption of nutrients is a problem because the food is not being broken down adequately to enable its absorption into the blood stream. The same is true when the colon is dysfunctional. Irritable bowel syndrome is a common complaint of individuals with fibromyalgia. Alternating diarrhea and constipation can be from abnormal colon function which then affects the nutritional status of all cells of the body.

Certain foods, vitamins, or allergies to foods or chemicals do not cause fibromyalgia. Individuals may find specific foods that appear to exacerbate symptoms and others that appear to help. In general, any food or drink that is an irritant to the nervous system may exacerbate symptoms. For example, the caffeine in coffee, tea, soda and chocolate is a nervous system irritant and aggravates symptoms of muscle pain, sleep disturbance, and bladder irritability. On the other hand, food or drink that has a quieting affect may help decrease symptoms. For example, the high fiber in complex carbohydrates may quiet irritable bowel symptoms.

Adequate consumption of water and noncaffeinated fluids is important for an FMS individual's health. The increased accumulation of waste products in muscle and connective tissues increases pain. Adequate fluid consumption, 6-8 glasses per day, helps the circulatory system and kidneys process waste products.

As described in Chapter 3, FMS research reports decreased amounts of chemical messengers like serotonin and norepinephrine which are composed of amino acid chains. There are several ways to potentially increase the levels of these chemical messengers. These include:

- boost their production through vitamin and mineral supplements
- increase the consumption of protein
- add amino acids supplements to the diet.

No one vitamin, mineral or amino acid can function on its own. It takes a group process to accomplish the manufacture and distribution of the chemical messengers that regulate the body. The most important amino acids that help to form the chemical messengers include:

- L-tyrosine,
- L-phenylalanine, and
- L-tryptophan.

The precursor to serotonin is L-tryptophan. The precursors to norepinephrine are L-tyrosine and L-phenlyalanine. Vitamin B6 is especially important because it directs development of the chemical messenger necklaces of amino acids. Sugar is important to avoid because it competes with amino acids for absorption in the intestines. Increased sugar intake can result in decrease amino acid absorption for use in the chemical messengers' necklaces.

There are many kinds and brands of amino acids on the market. It is important to use the "free form" type of amino acid supplement so they are ready to be used by the body without complicated digestion processes. The pharmaceutical grade of amino acids is the desired grade. It can be taken in a powder or capsule.

Some FMS individuals try to eat fatigue and achiness away. A common thought is, "If I just eat something I'll have more energy and not hurt as much." In other instances, when feelings of despair or depression are prevalent, the idea that food is a comforter leads to excessive calorie consumption. It is true that food can be quieting and comforting. Carbohydrates, for instance, tend to soothe the nervous system and gut. Yet it is important to recognize the symptoms and treat the pain, fatigue or depression, not try to cover them up or numb the senses with food.

It is vital to eat and drink adequately while exercising. Before starting an exercise program eat a light carbohydrate meal and drink 6-8 oz. of fluid. During workouts drink fluids every 10-15 minutes. It is important to consume a carbohydrate and protein meal within 15-20 minutes after exercise to replenish energy stores.

There are indications of decreased levels of magnesium in blood or muscle cells in FMS individuals. Five to eight hundred milligrams of magnesium daily is recommended by some experts.

Vitamins and minerals that are important in a daily dietary plan for FMS include:

Vitamin C – 500 to 3000 mg/day
Vitamin B Complex – 25-50 mg/day
Calcium – 800-1000 mg/day for females premenopause,
        1200-1500 mg/day menopause or post menopause
        (300 mg = 8 oz. milk or 1 slice cheese)
Vitamin E – 200-400 IU/day
Vitamin D – 20 minutes of sunlight/day
Malic Acid – 1200-1400 mg/day
Magnesium – 500-800 mg/day
(See Vitamin/Mineral Chart on page 118-119.)
Six to eight glasses of water daily! (decaffeinated fluids)

Vitamin/Mineral	Symptoms	Food Source
Vitamin B1	Fatigue	Wheat Germ
	Irritability	Brewer's Yeast
	Memory Loss	Soybeans
	Insomnia	Nuts
	Muscle Weakness	Poultry
	Numbness	Milk
	Tingling	
	Headaches	
	Increased Sensitivity to Pain	
	Heart Palpitations	
Vitamin B5	Fatigue	Organ Meats
	Muscle Weakness	Peanuts
	Muscle Cramps	Wheat Germ
	Hypoglycemia	Eggs
	Constipation	Beans
	Diarrhea	Peas

Vitamin/Mineral	Symptoms	Food Source
Vitamin B6	Irritability	Brewer's Yeast
	Insomnia	Liver
	Dizziness	Salmon
	PMS	Nuts
	Muscle Weakness	Brown Rice
	Numbness	Meats
	Tingling	Fish
	Hair Loss	Soybeans
	Hypoglycemia	
Vitamin B12	Mental Apathy	Liver
	Muscle Weakness	Egg Yolk
	Fatigue	Sardines
	Depression	Salmon
	Memory Loss	Crab
	Noise and Light Sensitivity	
	Chest Pain	
Vitamin C	Muscle Weakness	Broccoli
	Fatigue	Brussel Sprouts
	Confusion	Kale
	Joint Aches	Parsley
	Bruising	Green Peppers
	Poor Digestion	Rose Hips
	Infections	Lemons, Oranges.
		Tomatoes, Spinach,
		Cauliflower
Vitamin E	Muscle Pain	Vegetable Oils
	Muscle Weakness	Cottonseed
	PMS	Corn
	Decreased Circulation	Soybean, Nuts
	Infections	Legumes
	Leg Pain	
	Incoordination	
Magnesium	Fatigue	Wheat Germ
	Insomnia	Almonds
	Anxiety	Cashews
	Hyperactivity	Brazil Nuts
	Anger	Soybeans
	Tremors	Parsnips
	Numbness	Oats
	Tingling	Rye
	Rapid Pulse	Corn
	High Blood Pressure	
	Heart Irregularities	
Calcium	High Blood Pressure	Milk Products
	Osteoporosis	Cheese
	Muscle Pain	Yogurt
	Muscle Spasms	Canned Salmon
	Insomnia	Green Leafy Vegetables
	Nervousness	
	Hyperactivity	
	PMS	
Malic Acid	Muscle Pain	Apples
	Stiffness	Fruits

Vitamin C is present in citrus fruits and functions as an antioxidant, it may have antibiotic-like qualities at higher doses, and assists the intestines in normal functioning. Vitamin B complex, present in green leafy vegetables, is essential for nerve transmission and healthy functioning of the nerves and liver. It affects sleep, mental capacity, heart and lung functions. Vitamin E, present in brown rice, kale, apricots, sunflower and pumpkin seeds, can improve circulation and cellular function. Magnesium, present in green leafy vegetables, legumes and nuts, is essential for muscle and heart functioning. It inhibits action of excitatory amino acids that lead to increased pain and discomfort. Magnesium levels are inversely related to pain/tenderness levels, the higher the magnesium levels in muscle cells, the lower the pain complaints. Calcium, present in milk products, is essential for muscle function as well as bone strength. Calcium-magnesium combination is an effective muscle relaxant and sleep inducer. Malic acid is a food acid present in apples and other fruits. It is important for cell function and energy production in cells. It can be obtained as magnesium malate. Vitamin B12, if deficient, can cause fatigue and anemia.

It is possible to swallow all the right nutrients but unless the stomach and intestines are able to digest the nutrients and allow optimal absorption into the bloodstream the nutrients cannot benefit the individual. The enteric nervous system directs the function of the stomach and intestines. With dysfunction of the enteric nervous system common in FMS there is often abnormal nutrient absorption. Self care and medications that normalize the enteric nervous system and gut function can lead to significantly less fatigue and pain. Foods and supplements that are more completely digested will make a difference in pain and fatigue as well. Fructose based vitamin and mineral supplements have been the most effective for some FMS individuals. Any supplement should break down in water within 20 minutes to be effectively digested in the gut. Some FMS individuals utilize nutrients better if food combining strategies are followed, such as eating protein and vegetables together or avoiding protein and starches in combination.

Exercise

Exercise is the second step of general self stabilization. Exercise in moderation is essential to optimum function for FMS individuals. Moderate aerobic exercise, 20-30 minutes per day, is recommended.

Continue on the General Self Care Self Stabilizng Loop until all items are integrated into your daily life. Exercise guidelines are described in Chapter 20.

Medications

Medications are often recommended as part of the total management approach for FMS. Medications rarely eliminate all symptoms but often help with the sleep disorder and to decrease pain. To find the optimum medication combination, it may take the physician several trials of different medications in different amounts. Medication can be effective over an extended period. Medication may also lose its effectiveness after a period of time and need to be changed for another. Know what characteristics each medication has, its side effects, and how and when it should be taken. If there is more than one physician prescribing medication be sure that each physician knows all the medications being taken to avoid possible drug interactions. There are prescription guides available in bookstores or at the pharmacy to help you stay informed.

One last word about medication. Since FMS is a chronic condition, medications that help are frequently needed over an extended period of time and on a daily basis. There is a tendency for FMS individuals to take medication until they feel better and then quit taking it or take it infrequently. "I don't want to be dependent on drugs to feel good. I'm not someone who uses drugs," are commonly heard comments. The mind set that is needed when thinking about FMS and medications is that the individual has a lack of certain chemicals that then increase the fatigue and pain. The medications help replace those missing chemicals so the body can function optimally. They are often needed over the long term to help the FMS individual experience the fewest symptoms. Medication is one of the many tools an individual with FMS can use to help manage the symptoms of the illness and speed recovery. Stopping medications abruptly because of fears about drug use can cause a setback in treatment that is demoralizing. Medicine is not a crutch, it is an aid to ensuring improvement and should be respected as much as biofeedback or an exercise program. If an individual fears medication it is important to talk with the physician about the concerns.

Dress

The clothing a person wears makes a statement about personal style, helps with temperature regulation and offers protection. The FMS individual benefits from layered clothing so pieces can be added or subtracted as temperature changes. Air conditioning often increases FMS symptoms so light turtle necks and long sleeve shirts or sweaters are needed for protection in that environment. During winter weather silk or other light weight but warm underwear is often needed under all types of clothing. Glove and boot warmers are helpful if the person is going to be out in the cold weather. Tight, binding clothing is not tolerated when FMS symptoms include skin hypersensitivity or tender point pain in an area. Soft fabrics, elasticized waists, and sports bras will be more comfortable than tight, form fitting items. Supportive, well fitting shoes rather than slip on, high heel shoes are essential for daily life and the work environment. Walking or running shoes that have maximum cushioning are usually the best. Warm socks or slippers instead of bare feet are best at home.

Self Talk – Positive Self Statements

The mind is always saying something positive, negative, or neutral as an individual goes through the day. Even while sleeping at night there are thoughts and dreams. Self talk can be helpful or hurtful in relation to FMS symptoms and an individual's accomplishments. To develop an awareness of what self talk is like, for one or two days pause four or five times during the day and jot down what thoughts are present at that time in relation to what you are doing and how you are feeling. Are there primarily positive or negative thoughts? Are there repetitive thoughts? Now take the positive thoughts and repeat them throughout the day such as every time breathing practice is scheduled or every time you talk on the phone. Pair the positive self statement with some event that occurs frequently in the day. If there is negative self talk, substitute positive statements for the negative thoughts.

Examples of positive self statements are:

- I am healing, I am healing more each moment of each day.
- I am trying, I am doing the best I can.
- I deserve to be healthy and happy, I am healthy and happy.
- I feel quiet and calm, I am quiet and calm.
- I love you, I will take care of you.

For some individuals positive self statements seem like lies or half truths. If that occurs, put "I am trying" or "I am beginning to" in front of the statement. Remember every thought stimulates biochemical and electrical events in the brain and gut which then flow to every cell of the body and affect all other body and mind functions.

Rest is a Treatment Essential in FMS

Rest is a vital part of anyone's daily schedule, usually accomplished at an unconscious level. Relaxing into a chair for a few minutes between jobs, reading the newspaper or watching television and dozing off for a short period, sitting under a tree and gazing at the clouds during lunch time, or sitting at your desk stretching towards the ceiling while releasing two or three big sighs are all forms of rest the body and mind need and ask for throughout the day. Rest is necessary for energy conservation and a return to neutrality and slow idle before going on to a new task.

Both mind and body rest are important to accomplish during the slow idle periods throughout the day. Mind rest techniques can include meditation, positive self talk, and breathing awareness to name a few. Body rest includes skeletal muscle release and internal organ systems' quieting using Physiological Quieting techniques such as breathing and hand warming. The need for supportive, comfortable chairs, couches and beds that enable the individual's muscles to let go into a relaxed state with minimal pain are important for body rest.

Mind and body rest needs to occur frequently throughout the day for short periods. Sometimes it will only be a minute or so of breathing and quiet muscle release, other times 5 minutes of focused meditation, and at least 20-30 minutes of extended mind and body rest using Physiological Quieting techniques once a day. When setting up a schedule for the day, **rest periods are as important as work periods**. These rest periods help ensure that the FMS tendency for elevated resting levels of muscle activity, autonomic nervous system activity and mental activity are frequently returned to more normal levels, to a slow idle. These rest periods can be essential in maintaining a decreased pain and fatigue level throughout the day instead of the pattern of a small window of relief in the morning with escalating pain and fatigue levels for the remainder of the day.

Pacing – Energy Management

Pacing is the breaking up of the day into multiple work, rest, and play sections. To pace the day it is important to first make a list of the work related tasks for the day and prioritize the top three while putting the others off until tomorrow. Pacing is breaking each of those jobs or tasks into two or three parts with planned rest periods in between.

Pacing is never finishing one job before you start a part of another one. Instead it means performing the first part of job one, then resting, then going to the first part of job two, then resting, then completing the first part of job three, then resting, then going back to the second part of job one, etc. With this kind of pacing, different muscles and different body postures are used for each new job. Fatigue is less of a problem because parts of jobs are done with frequent changes in muscle action and postural alignment. Frequent short rest periods with conscious return to neutral mind and body activity enables the FMS individual to accomplish more tasks with less fatigue and pain.

Daily Job List

1. Sweep floors
2.
3.
4.
5.
6.
7.

Daily Priority Jobs

1. Sweep floors
   a. part one: Sweep 1/2 kitchen floor
   b. part two: Sweep 1/2 kitchen floor
   c. part three: Sweep laundry room
2.
   a. part one:
   b. part two:
   c. part three:
3.
   a. part one:
   b. part two:
   c. part three:

Rest Activities

- Listening to music while reclining.
- Reading in supported sitting.
- Physiological Quieting.
- Meditation

Initially the rest cycles may be longer than work cycles, but gradually the two will become equal and eventually the work cycle can exceed the rest cycle and still maintain the goals of decreased pain and fatigue. For example:

Rest Cycle	Work Cycle
10 minutes	3-5 minutes
	increase 1-2 minutes/week
10 minutes	10 minutes
10 minutes	15 minutes

Play and Fun

Pacing means placing play and laughter into the work-rest routine throughout the day, not just when all work has been accomplished. **Play and laughter are required treatments multiple times during each day.** With that being the case, short periods of play will be scheduled into mid morning, mid afternoon, and evening. On some occasions, segments can be as simple and short as reading the funnies in the paper every morning and making sure to practice belly laughing. There needs to be a daily 20-30 minute play period with friends over tea, or spending 20 minutes in a hot bath or hot tub, going to the movie, or watching a favorite TV program.

Some individuals, when asked what they do for fun, respond "work." It is necessary to begin making a master list of play and fun activities that are not work related so you can vary the play activities on a daily and weekly basis and continue to be on the lookout for a new play or fun activity to add to the list. Try to find a new one every week or two. Watch other people and catch them having fun, see what they are doing. It means that play and laughter have equal weight with work and rest in a daily schedule.

Pacing of work, rest and play can be easily monitored by using a daily journal. As part of a nightly routine fill in the day's activities and summarize where pacing went well.

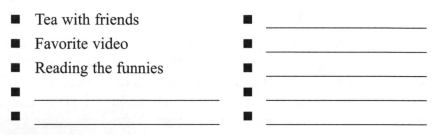

DAILY JOURNAL OF PLAY, REST, WORK

Date_____

Time	Play	Rest	Work
			(ea. task = 3 parts) (3-4 tasks/day)
A.M. 7:00-8:00			
8:00-9:00			
9:00-10:00			

Play Activity List

- Tea with friends
- Favorite video
- Reading the funnies
- _____
- _____

- _____
- _____
- _____
- _____
- _____

Prioritizing

Prioritizing is making decisions – decisions that some work is more important to do today, that some work is more important to do next week and some work you should never do but rather give to someone else or let it go undone. Prioritizing is listing all the work titles you have and the roles you carry out under each of those, then making decisions as to which are important to be done on a daily, weekly, monthly or never ever basis. It needs to be emphasized that prioritizing is done in the context of the pacing schedule you have already planned. **Prioritizing is more important than getting all your work roles accomplished. Figure out how the work roles can fit into your optimum pacing schedule.**

Work Titles I Fulfill	**Roles**
	Examples:
■ Parent to children	■ Transporter
■ Parent to elderly parents (list specifics)	■ House cleaner
■ Spouse	■ Listener/emotional support
■ Banker, teacher, teller etc.	■ Money transfer, reaching, grasp
■ Volunteer	
■ Friend	

Pain Relieving Modalities

Pain relief is the number one priority for most individuals with fibromyalgia. Effective techniques may be different for each person. Examples of pain relieving modalities include:

Heat

The benefits from 20-30 minutes of heat include increased circulation and decreased muscle tightness. Moist heat pads are usually preferred over dry heating pads. The moist heating pad purchased at the drug store will often have little sponges that are moistened. Medical supply stores have heating pads that draw moisture from the air. They are a little more costly but are larger and conform better to the body contours. A damp towel or commercial hot pack heated in the microwave or in hot water for a few minutes is another good way to get moist heat. Hot water in the form of a hot tub, hot shower, or whirlpool bath is always a good choice. Hot tubs need to be under $102°$ F to allow an individual to stay in the water comfortably and safely for 20-30 minutes.

Cold

Some individuals benefit from ice so it is worth a try even if it sounds uncomfortable. One form of treatment is an ice massage to a painful area. Freeze water in an 8 oz. paper cup, then tear away the top edge of paper so the ice can be moved around the palm size painful area for about five minutes. Initially it feels very cold but within five minutes the area will be numb. Use a towel to catch the drips. Some individuals find it more tolerable to use ice while in a hot tub or shower or while they have heat on another part of the body. If cold hands are a problem, use gloves and a styrofoam cup.

An ice pack is another form of cold application. Commercial ice packs and ice probes are available through medical supply stores. Ice packs can be homemade using a wet or dry towel wrapped around a package of frozen peas or corn or crushed ice. A frozen wet towel provides more intense cold. A ten minute application of an ice pack is usually adequate.

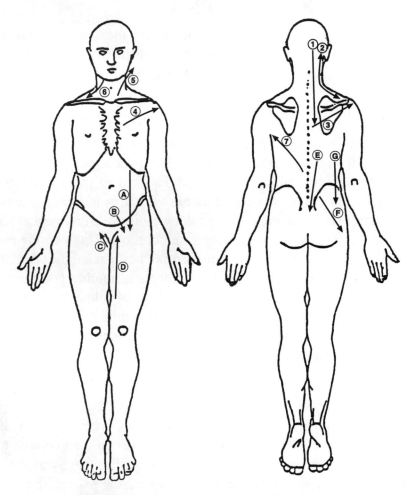

Figure 12: Vapocoolant Spray Techniques

Cold Spray – Heat

This technique is designed to obtain effective pain relief and increased motion in affected body areas. Vapocoolant spray is a cold, fine spray of gas under pressure. It is prescribed by a physician for clinic and/or home use. At home it is initially used for 7-10 days to decrease symptoms and then it is used as needed during acute exacerbations or after exercise. For use with FMS, body segments are treated instead of one or two specific muscles and the body position during the treatment is more midline than stretched as it is when myofascial muscle shortening is being treated. The term "midline spray and heat" is used rather than the more common term "spray and stretch." Initially a physician or therapist can use the technique as part of the office visit to evaluate effectiveness and improve pain and limited range of motion. If the technique is effective, the health care professional can demonstrate the techniques to a support person so a home program can be done 1-2 times daily during painful flare-ups (Figure 12). When pain is primarily in the upper body, (neck, shoulders, arms, shoulder blades, chest) the spray techniques 1-7 are completed bilaterally even though the pain and limited range of motion are present on only one side. When pain is primarily in the lower body, (low back, hips, buttocks, legs, abdomen) the spray techniques A-G are completed bilaterally.

Alternate – Heat – Ice

Some individuals get the most benefit from using a combination of heat and ice. Use heat (heating pad, hot tub) for 7-10 minutes, then cold (ice pack, ice probe) for 3-5 minutes, and then heat for 7-10 minutes.

Heat – Stretch and Ice – Heat

This technique is designed to obtain an effective stretch of a tight muscle group without setting off muscle spasms. Heat the muscle group for about three minutes, then put that area on a gentle stretch and hold the stretch while rubbing an ice cup or ice edge in lines about 1/2 inch apart parallel to the muscle fibers under the skin. Keep the stretch gentle and steady for 30-60 seconds then heat the area again for approximately three minutes.

Oils and Lotions

A number of lotions, creams and oils can be used in combination with medication to ease muscle pain and tightness. Especially for those individuals who are drug sensitive, oils and lotions don't cause stomach or gastrointestinal irritation or the side effects of some medications yet they can give relief from pain and muscle tightness.

Essential oil mixtures in a base oil such as almond oil can be easily applied to painful areas by the individual or family member. Specific oils decrease pain, detoxify waste products and improve circulation. Commonly used essential oils include lavender, lemon, rosemary, juniper, and bergamot. See Product Sources on page 229.

Lotions containing capsaicin are known to decrease substance P. Capsaicin is derived from red peppers and produces a hot, burning sensation when rubbed into the skin. Repeated application to a specific area over a week can result in decreased pain. Other lotions produce a cooling effect on the skin for relief of pain and discomfort.

Massage

Self massage or having a family member massage areas can be effective using essential oils and light to moderate stroking over muscle areas that are painful or tight. The touch helps quiet and relax the muscles and the essential oils help increase circulation, decrease pain and tightness. It is important to avoid trying to "dig out" the pain with deep, intense massage techniques which will often increase the symptoms. The pain does not have to get worse before it can get better. Tender point pressure, direct pressure using the thumb or a finger for 7-8 seconds, is one beneficial technique. Direct pressure over acupressure sites for 7-8 seconds can be effective for pain relief and easy to do several times a day (Figure 13).

To reach hard to get areas use two tennis balls in a sock and place the balls between the individual and the floor to massage a particular spot for 1-3 minutes to decrease pain. Two racket balls in a sock fit the base of the neck better than tennis balls. There are various canes and knobs on the market to help you reach difficult spots. Hiring a professional massage therapist for a weekly massage is also beneficial. Interview them first, to make sure they understand the needs of fibromyalgia.

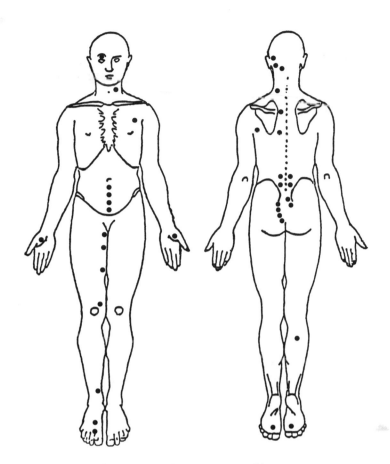

Figure 13: Acupressure Sites

Journaling

The habit of regularly writing in a blank book or on pages in a notebook can be helpful in tracking the ups and downs of fibromyalgia, in seeing small steps of progress that lead to improved health, and in relieving the "free floating" anxiety FMS individuals describe.

Journaling is "stream of conscious" writing. There is no right or wrong way to do it. Just open the blank book or take some note paper and write whatever flows from the mind and hand. No one needs to read it or judge it. Let the mind empty all its thoughts, worries, and concerns on the paper. When the censor part of the mind tries to stop the thought flow to the paper, remember this writing is not for judging, it is for releasing feeling and thoughts.

In FMS at times the brain activity for thoughts, worries, and ideas becomes excessive, getting in the way of everyday life just as the muscles become overactive causing pain and fatigue. The overactive brain leads to feelings of anxiety, confusion, indecision, and mental paralysis. Releasing any and all thoughts to paper assists in quieting brain activity.

Journaling can be done day or night. Keep notebooks on a bed stand and in a purse. Some FMS individuals are not able to write so a computer or audio or video tape recorder is a better mode of communication.

A second type of daily journal is designed to give a picture of patterns and relationships between symptoms, work, exercise, rest, and sleep. On a longitudinal 24 hour scale the FMS individual keeps track of pain levels, sleep hours, number of awakenings at night, work, rest, and exercise cycles. See the Weekly Self Care Report on page 133. Progress or problems can be seen more easily with this type of journaling.

It can be helpful to keep a daily journal to pick up patterns and relationships between symptoms and daily activities and stressors. In the journal the FMS individual keeps track of pain, stiffness and fatigue levels during morning, noon, afternoon and evening, medication taken, menstrual cycle pattern, exercise level, and jobs done.

The goal for FMS individuals is to modify activities or stressors that increase symptoms so there is an equilibrium achieved for extended periods of time. The equilibrium is often not a completely pain-free state, nor totally fatigue-free, but interventions throughout the day keep the equilibrium. A self care routine with regular mini reassessments of mind-body function are essential to attain that steady state of equilibrium.

Crisis Management Program

Flare-ups or exacerbations are going to occur in FMS even with the best management program. A prearranged crisis management plan will help the FMS individual deal with the flare-ups. The crisis management plan is comprised of items that have worked in the past in order of priority, a list of support people to contact, and positive self statements that direct the mind and body towards health and healing.

WEEKLY SELF CARE REPORT

Record your symptoms and activities according to the following guidelines.
Rate your **pain** 4x/day on a scale of 0 to 10. 0=no pain 10= excruciating pain.
Indicate **rest periods** using **R**. Indicate **exercises** using **E**,
Indicate **play periods** using **P**.
Indicate **hours slept** and **number of awakenings** in the parenthesis.

See the following example.

Date: **6/15/00**

6	R	5	E	7	6	(7/5)
awaken		lunch		dinner	bed	

Comments:_____

Date:_____

						( )
awaken		lunch		dinner	bed	

Comments:_____

Date:_____

						( )
awaken		lunch		dinner	bed	

Comments:_____

Date:_____

						( )
awaken		lunch		dinner	bed	

Comments:_____

Date:_____

						( )
awaken		lunch		dinner	bed	

Comments:_____

Date:_____

						( )
awaken		lunch		dinner	bed	

Comments:_____

Date:_____

						( )
awaken		lunch		dinner	bed	

Comments:_____

Date:_____

						( )
awaken		lunch		dinner	bed	

Comments:_____

Examples of Crisis Management Plan

Alter the day's plans to fit your needs!

- Use modalities such as hot shower or hot tub for 20 minutes.
- Take 20 minutes 2-3 times today for Physiological Quieting.
- Use pain relieving oil or lotion on affected muscles.
- . Do breathing and hand warming every half hour to hour.
- Take a relaxing walk with a friend.
- Take medication as directed for crisis times.
- Increase rest cycle length in the daily plan.
- Emphasize positive self statements.
- Evaluate life stressors, i.e., environmental, emotional.
- Consult with therapist or physician if not improved in 48 hours.

My Crisis Management Plan

1. _____

2. _____

3. _____

4. _____

5. _____

What Can I Do To Manage Fibromyalgia Through Subcategory Self Stabilizing Loops?

An Overview

	Characteristics	Test	Treatment
Type **1** a General Hypoglycemic Tendencies	symptoms 2-3 hrs. post meal, shaky, weak, irritable, irrational, confused, relieved by complex carbohydrate intake	Blood Glucose Monitoring	Complex Carbos 5-6 meals/day Exercise
Type **1** b Reactive Hypoglycemic Tendencies	symptoms 20-30 min. post meal, shaky, weak, low blood sugar, irritable, irrational, confused, relieved by protein & fat intake	Blood Glucose Monitoring	Incr. Fat & Protein 5-6 meals/day Exercise
Type **2** Hypothyroid Tendencies	dry skin, thinning hair, cold, constipation, muscle ache, fatigue, weight gain	Basal Body Temp	L Tyrosine Kelp Exercise
Type **3** Neurally Mediated Hypotension Tendencies	low blood pressure, high resting heart rate disequilibrium, dizzy, weak, abdominal pain	Blood Pressure Heart Rate Tilt Table Test	Salt Pool Exercise
Type **4** Reproductive Hormonal Imbalance	cyclical symptoms related to hormonal cycle in females, severe sleep disturbance	History Hormonal Levels	DHEA Phyto Hormones Exercise
Type **5** Immune System Imbalance	fatigue, diarrhea, muscle pain, confusion	Immune System Questionnaire	Acidophilus Low Sugar Co Enzyme Q Vitamin B12

Treatment Guidelines for Fibromyalgia

🄖 General Guidelines

- Sleep Protocol
- Nutrition Protocol
- Exercise Protocol
- Physiological Quieting Protocol
- Positive Self Statement/ Journaling Protocol
- Modality Protocol
- Work/Rest Pacing Protocol

1 a Hypoglycemic Tendencies

- eliminate refined sugars, fruit juice, white flour
- increase complex carbohydrates
- eat frequent, small meals- every 3 hours
- vitamins/minerals
    - chromium picolinate 300-600mcg.
    - vitamin B complex 50-100mg.
    - coenzyme Q 25-50mg.   • zinc 50mg.
- herbs
    - bilberry   • wild yam
- exercise 30 min. daily, moderate aerobic
- Physiological Quieting 20 min. daily

1 b Reactive Hypoglycemic Tendencies

- eliminate refined sugars, fruit juice, white flour
- increase fat and protein
    - Zone Diet   • 40% carbohydrates, 30% protein, 30% fat
- begin the day with fat to set the ileal brake
- eat frequent, small meals every 2 hours
- vitamins/minerals
    - vitamin B complex 50-100mg.
    - chromium picolinate 300-600mcg.
    - coenzyme Q 20-50mg.   • zinc 50mg.
- herbs
    - bilberry   • wild yam
- exercise 30 min daily, moderate aerobic
- Physiological Quieting 20 min. daily

2 Hypothyroid Tendencies

- nutritional changes
  - kelp 1000-3000mg
  - vitamin B12 15-45mg
  - vitamin C 100mg
  - magnesium 400-800mg.
  - essential fatty acids (EFAs)
  - L-tyrosine 1000mg.
  - vitamin B6 50mg
  - malic acid 1200-1400mg
- avoid chlorine and fluoride
- exercise 30 min. daily moderate aerobic
- Physiological Quieting 20 min. daily

Chapter 17

3 Neurally Mediated Hypotension Tendencies

- nutritional changes
  - increase salt-sodium chloride
  - monitor magnesium levels
  - eliminate caffeine, refined sugars
  - increase fat and protein ratio to carbohydrates
  - increase foods with tryptophan
    - turkey, milk
  - increase gut quieting foods
    - rice, applesauce, bananas
  - assess gut intolerant foods
    - lactose (milk), wheat, MSG, spicy foods
- herbs
  - licorice
- positional draining of pelvic vericosities
  - hips higher than head
- essential oils
  - teas: peppermint, chamomile
  - external: angelica, balm, bergamot, clary, lavender, mint, neroli, orange and rose
- exercise 30 min. daily moderate aerobic
  - pool exercise shoulder height water

Chapter 13: What Can I Do To Manage Fibromyalgia Through
Self Stabilizing Subcategory Loops?

137

▉4 Immune System Dysregulation Tendencies

■ nutritional changes
  • eliminate refined sugars
  • acidophilus bacteria
  • caprylic acid &/or garlic capsules
  • coenzyme Q 25-50mg.
  • vitamin B12 14-45mg.
  • vitamin C 250-1000mg.
  • vitamin E 250mg.
  • essential fatty acids (EFAs)
■ herbs
  • echinacea
  • goldenseal
  • licorice
  • panax ginseng
■ exercise 30 min. daily moderate aerobic
■ Physiological Quieting 20-30 min. daily

▉5 Reproductive Hormone Dysregulation Tendencies

■ nutritional changes
  • phytoestrogen/progesterone foods
       soy, flax seed, green tea
  • eliminate caffeine and refined sugars
  • vitamin C 250-1000 mg
■ nonprescription creams or pills
  • phytoestrogen/progesterone
  • vitalaxin (oxytocin)
  • DHEA
■ exercise 30 min. daily moderate aerobic
■ Physiological Quieting 20 min. daily

138

Chapter 13: What Can I Do To Manage Fibromyalgia Through
Self Stabilizing Subcategory Loops?

Chapter 14

Research and Inquiry

The research to support self care interventions, specifically exercise and medication, is plentiful. Exercise, medication, daily rest-work cycles, and biofeedback have helped to decrease pain and fatigue. The research to support the management of FMS using the subcategory types is primarily clinical in nature. Hulme and Penner reported results in 200 females using self management in conjunction with medication. Before treatment, functional and work activity was greatly disrupted in 10% of the individuals, moderately disrupted in 79%, and minimally disrupted in 11%. Problems described included pain, stiffness, and fatigue with activity and associated symptoms. Treatment included lifetime strategies of self care in conjunction with medication, exercise, biofeedback and modalities. Seventy three percent of the 200 individuals reported improved pain levels and 65% increased daily functional work activity after 6 weeks of intervention. (Figure 14) Relief of associated symptoms had equal or greater impact on functional work activity levels compared to pain relief.

Exercise endurance increased with the lifetime strategies of self care from an average of 15 minutes (range 0-30 minutes) to 30 minutes (range 5-54 minutes).

When subcategory assessment and self care stabilizing loops were part of the treatment protocol, exercise endurance increased to an average of 45 minutes (15-60minutes). (Figure 15) This indicates that individuals with FMS can in many cases increase their exercise and daily activity endurance more with use of the subcategory types and subsequent interventions.

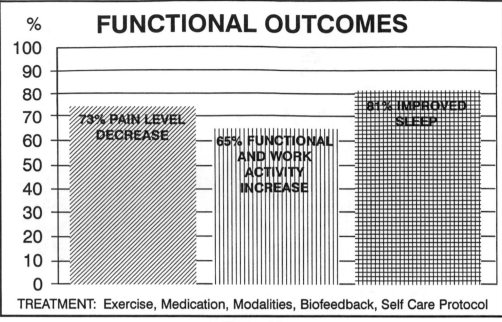

Figure 14

EXERCISE ENDURANCE

	BASELINE	REGULAR TREATMENT	ADD SUBSET TREATMENT
average minutes	15	30	45
range	0-30	5-45	15-60

Note: 15 minute increments without increase pain/fatigue

Figure 15

Chapter 15

1 Hypoglycemic Tendencies Self Stabilizing Loop

The Type 1 subcategory of fibromyalgia is termed hypoglycemic tendencies.

Symptoms

These individuals describe feeling shaky, dizzy, irritable, irrational and weak. Other symptoms include headache, depression, anxiety, sweets cravings, confusion, night sweats, and insomnia. These individuals can become aggressive and easily lose their tempers during a hypoglycemic episode. Stress increases the levels of stress hormones. Stress hormones increase metabolism, activate insulin release, and increase glucose utilization.

Even though the standard definition of hypoglycemia is a blood sugar level below 50mg/dl, in recent years there have been several studies that suggest individuals have different set points for blood sugar. When there is a drop below the individual's specific set point the brain and body exhibit "I'm in trouble" signs. The set point in the research studies varied from the 50s to the 80s. That means that an FMS individual could have a high set point in the 70s or 80s and exhibit symptoms of muscle stiffness, cramping and weakness, fatigue, irritability, insomnia, and mental confusion due to "hypoglycemic tendencies." The patient's history and symptoms will provide the best indication of this subtype of FMS although blood sugar levels can be of help if there is an acceptance that symptoms and set points are the criteria, not a blood glucose reading of 50.

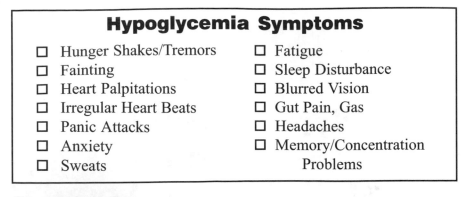

Hypoglycemia Symptoms

- ☐ Hunger Shakes/Tremors
- ☐ Fainting
- ☐ Heart Palpitations
- ☐ Irregular Heart Beats
- ☐ Panic Attacks
- ☐ Anxiety
- ☐ Sweats
- ☐ Fatigue
- ☐ Sleep Disturbance
- ☐ Blurred Vision
- ☐ Gut Pain, Gas
- ☐ Headaches
- ☐ Memory/Concentration Problems

Case Study

Linda's husband describes her as the sweetest, most giving person he has ever met yet he comments that she has a tendency to snap and blow up at any little thing. He notes that she frequently complains of pain in her shoulders, neck and head. She sometimes wakes him up at night in a sweat. These symptoms began after the birth of their first child so they assumed it was just a readjustment from pregnancy. Now two years later they are both concerned that the symptoms haven't gone away. Her physician diagnosed fibromyalgia and the medications have helped some but she still experiences fatigue, pain, and mood changes that have a rapid onset, i.e. one minute she's feeling good and the next she feels lousy.

Etiology/Cause

Hypoglycemia is a condition of low blood glucose (sugar) levels with resulting symptoms. Any or all of the symptoms may occur as quickly as 30-60 minutes after a meal or as long as 2-3 hours after eating. For some reason there is an imbalance between insulin and glucose in the blood stream which leads to the low blood sugar.

The two subtypes of hypoglycemia are:

- ■ General Hypoglycemia
- ■ Reactive Hypoglycemia

The two subtypes are differentiated by 1) the time frame between eating and the onset of low blood sugar and 2) the type of food that sets off the symptoms. In General Hypoglycemia the onset of hypoglycemic symptoms is usually 2-3 hours after a meal. In Reactive Hypoglycemia the onset of symptoms is more immediate, usually 30-60 minutes after eating. In the case of General Hypoglycemia the foods that set off the symptoms include simple sugars and carbohydrates but not complex carbohydrates. In the case of Reactive Hypoglycemia complex carbohydrates as well as simple sugars and carbohydrates can set off the symptoms.

- General Hypoglycemia   2-3 hrs. simple sugars/carbos
- Reactive Hypoglycemia   1/2-1 hr. complex carbos
                                       simple sugars/carbos

Both the time between eating and symptoms and the type of food eaten relate to the release of insulin and glucose (sugar) into the blood stream. This model for hypoglycemia takes into consideration the timing of insulin release from the pancreas and the timing of glucose release from the small intestine. The model also takes into consideration the amount of insulin or glucose released within a set amount of time, it could be a large amount (bolus) released in a short time period or smaller amounts (timed release capsules) over a 3-4 hour segment.

- General Hypoglycemia   Bolus insulin and glucose released in 1-2 hours symptoms experienced
- Reactive Hypoglycemia   Premature bolus of insulin released Timed released glucose 1/2-1 hour symptoms experienced

In both hypoglycemia subtypes simple sugars/carbohydrates stimulate excessive movement of insulin and glucose into the blood stream (the sugar high) depleting the glucose available in a short amount of time. The result is low blood sugar (the crash). In reactive hypoglycemia complex carbohydrates also stimulate excessive and premature release of insulin. In both hypoglycemia subtypes stress, excessive exercise, caffeine or alcohol can stimulate hypoglycemic symptoms.

This cause of General Hypoglycemia is based on a dysfunctional glucose absorption model. Glucose is absorbed abnormally from the small intestine into the blood stream. The small intestine is the primary area of the gastrointestinal tract where nutrients are absorbed. If sugars are absorbed more slowly than insulin is released, low blood sugar results – hypoglycemia. The blood sugar and insulin are not balanced in the blood stream. The enteric nervous system controls sugar absorption from the gut to the blood stream and release of insulin from the pancreas. When the enteric brake is "on" the gut slows or even stops the absorption of nutrients into the blood stream. When the enteric brake is "off" the gut speeds up the absorption of nutrients into the blood stream. The enteric brake is stimulated to be "off" when sugars and simple carbohydrates enter the stomach. In General Hypoglycemia the enteric brake is "off" so the gut sends sugars to the blood stream and the pancreas sends insulin into the blood stream more rapidly than normal. Within a 2-3 hour period the available glucose is utilized and blood sugar levels drop. The FMS individual with general hypoglycemic tendencies exhibits symptoms that interfere with their daily life when blood sugar levels drop into the 70/80 range or below.

The cause of Reactive Hypoglycemia is based on an abnormal insulin release model. Insulin is released prematurely and excessively by the pancreas. In Reactive Hypoglycemia, when simple or complex carbohydrates are chewed and swallowed, the enteric nervous system sends messages to the pancreas telling it to immediately release insulin into the bloodstream at a rapid rate and in substantial amounts. Meanwhile, back in the gut, the carbohydrate is taking hours to be digested and then absorbed into the bloodstream. The insulin looks for the great quantity of sugar (glucose) that the enteric nervous system said would be waiting for it in the bloodstream and finds relatively little. It combines with any glucose it finds but soon runs out of available glucose. The imbalance of insulin versus glucose in the bloodstream leads to a rapid depletion of blood glucose resulting in the symptoms of shakiness, confusion, pain, fatigue and agitation within 30-60 minutes of eating. The organ systems i.e., the brain, muscles, blood vessels are not getting the consistent level of glucose combined with insulin they need to function normally.

The Tortoise and the Hare

An analogy with a running race may help describe hypoglycemia even more effectively. In a race the participants (the pancreas and the intestines) are lined up at the starting blocks ready to take off at the sound of the starter's gun. In the case of General Hypoglycemia the pancreas and intestines are both hyper-alert if simple sugars and carbos have been eaten before the race. They take off too fast depleting all their stores of energy before the end of the race (the next scheduled meal). They cannot complete the race except by crawling or getting a ride.

In the case of Reactive Hypoglycemia one racer (the pancreas) notices the starter (the enteric nervous system) twitch or cough and prematurely takes off in a false start. The intestines do not false start, they may even be slow to start in confusion over the false start. The pancreas depletes the available store of energy too quickly and the intestines have not effectively released their energy store to even get in the race.

Testing

The first assessment is a review of symptoms by the individual and a close family member or friend (See Symptoms, Page 142). The involvement of a family member or friend is important because the individual may not be aware of all the external appearances of symptoms if the hypoglycemia is moderate to severe. Individuals with long term hypoglycemia may assume the symptoms are normal feelings.

When the symptom review is completed the next step is to monitor blood glucose levels periodically throughout the day for 1-2 days. It is important to also keep track of the food eaten at each meal and snack and any symptoms you are experiencing at the time of the blood glucose reading. Blood glucose readings every hour or two can indicate General or Reactive Hypoglycemic tendencies. In both conditions take blood glucose readings:

- on awakening each morning
- prior to each meal
- 1 hour after each meal
- 3 hours after each meal if another meal has not been eaten
- prior to going to bed

Optimal blood glucose range is 90-120. Below 90 individuals can begin to experience symptoms and by the time an individual reaches 80 they describe feeling significant symptoms. In the 60-70 range work and self care function is severely affected.

To determine which subtype of hypoglycemia is present monitor the blood glucose readings after a high carbohydrate meal and then after a high protein/fat meal. Assess how quickly the symptoms occur after eating. Fatigue, pain and personality changes within 30 minutes to one hour after eating a high carbohydrate meal is more likely Reactive Hypoglycemia. Fatigue, pain and personality changes 2-3 hours after a meal relatively high in simple sugars/carbohydrates is more likely General Hypoglycemia.

It is important to test immediately on awakening and as you go to bed each night. Hypoglycemia can occur at night as well as during the day. If blood sugar is low as you go to bed at night and/or low when you first wake up in the morning the implication is that you are experiencing hypoglycemic tendencies during the night. Sleep disturbance and night sweats are common with night time hypoglycemia.

A glucose tolerance test (GTT) performed in a medical center can indicate hypoglycemia. The individual is required to fast for 12 hours and then glucose is given in measured doses. The test is usually done over 5 hours testing the level of glucose in the blood each hour. If glucose levels are low or erratic the diagnosis is made of hypoglycemia. Some individuals will have normal test results but still experience symptoms.

Case Study

Larry, a 45 year old plumber, describes having fibromyalgia for the past 4 years since an auto accident caused whiplash. On awakening in the morning he is stiff and sore so he immediately takes a hot shower and does some stretching to get ready for the day. His usual breakfast before going to work is a bowl of oatmeal with raisins and brown sugar, 2 slices of toast with butter and jam, a large glass of orange juice and 2 cups of coffee. His wife states he comes to the breakfast table in a good mood but after breakfast he usually has something nasty to say and sometimes forgets his keys and lunch box as he leaves. Larry says that after breakfast he feels more tired physically and mentally than before breakfast. He doesn't understand how that could be.

In Larry's case the high carbohydrate breakfast stimulated an immediate and large release of insulin into the blood stream. The carbohydrates are still primarily in the stomach while the insulin pours into the blood stream and combines with any glucose it can find. The result is the blood glucose levels drop significantly and quickly. Within 30 minutes Larry was feeling "lousy." He would go back to bed if he could.

Individuals like Larry tell us that when they ate steak and eggs for breakfast they all felt much better, have more energy and less pain, and an improved personality. Larry remembers times during the work day when he felt shaky and tired. If he stopped by McDonald's and got a Big Mac he felt better quickly. Was this just a break from work or did Big Macs have a miraculous quality? What should be bad to eat seemed to be good for Larry and others with fibromyalgia.

Treatment

General Hypoglycemic Tendencies

Symptoms of General Hypoglycemia decrease with the elimination of simple sugars in the diet and an increase in complex carbohydrate consumption. Whole grains and vegetables are recommended instead of candy bars and colas even though that is what the individual may crave. Consumption of fruit juice and white flour is not recommended. Whole fruits like apples can be consumed in moderation – 1-2 a day. Avocados tend to depress insulin production so hypoglycemic tendencies can be improved with the consumption of avocados. Reducing meat protein while increasing complex carbohydrates is beneficial. Consuming complex carbohydrates every 3 hours can provide a more stable blood glucose level so 6 small meals a day, or 3 meals and 3 snacks is a better plan than 3 meals a day spaced 4-5 hours apart. It is important that individuals with hypoglycemic tendencies eat a small carbohydrate meal before going to bed at night. This helps to maintain the blood glucose levels through the night.

Vitamins and minerals can be helpful in hypoglycemia regulation. Chromium picolinate 300-600 mcg, vitamin B complex 50-100 mg, and coenzyme Q can all assist in stabilizing blood sugar levels. Zinc, 50 mg daily, is needed for insulin release from the pancreas. Herbs that may help hypoglycemic tendencies include bilberry and wild yam.

Exercise in moderation can help to stabilize blood glucose levels if it is done on a daily basis and at the same level of exertion daily. In general, exercise assists in balancing the body's hormonal levels. More specifically, exercise can be beneficial in maintaining blood glucose levels because of more stable insulin levels.

Physiological Quieting has an important place in preventing hypoglycemic symptoms. Stress increases hypoglycemic tendencies in fibromyalgia. If stress becomes a chronic way of life the stress hormones are "used up" and these low levels of stress hormones result in insulin production changes.

---

1 a Self Care for General Hypoglycemia Tendencies

- Blood glucose testing multiple times/day
- Nutritional changes:
  - small meals every 2-3 hours
  - increase complex carbohydrates
  - refined sugars, fruit juice, white flour eliminated
  - vitamin/mineral boosters
    - chromium picolinate 300-600mcg
    - vitamin B complex 50-100mg
    - coenzyme Q 25-50mg   – zinc 50mg
  - herb booster
    - bilberry   – wild yam
- Exercise: moderate aerobic, 30 min/daily
- Physiological Quieting: 20-30 min/daily

Treatment

Reactive Hypoglycemic Tendencies

Symptoms of Reactive Hypoglycemic Tendencies decrease with an elimination of simple sugars in the diet and an increase in fat and protein. Protein and fat intake slows the release of insulin in Reactive Hypoglycemia. Proteins break down into amino acids in the gut. It takes a much longer time to break down protein to amino acids than it takes to break down carbohydrates to glucose/sugar molecules. Amino acids stimulate different enteric nervous system responses than carbohydrates and glucose. Therefore, eating a relatively high protein breakfast could prevent the reactive hypoglycemic symptoms of fatigue, confusion, agitation, and pain. Instead the individual feels energized for the rest of the day.

Fat, similar to protein, slows the release of insulin. Fats break down into fatty acids in the gut. It takes longer to break down fat into fatty acids than it does to break down carbohydrates to glucose/sugar. Fatty acids stimulate different enteric nervous system responses than carbohydrates and glucose do. Therefore eating a relatively high fat diet can prevent the reactive hypoglycemic symptoms of fatigue, confusion, agitation, and pain.

Both protein and fat tend to set the enteric brake "on" so the pancreas is stimulated to release insulin and the small intestine is stimulated to release nutrients into the blood stream in a more graded, gradual fashion.

Combining carbohydrate, protein, and fat in each meal in a 40%, 30%, 30% ratio provides the enteric nervous system of the gut with the needed balance for more normal insulin release throughout the day. There is a need to eat frequently, usually every 2 hours. The first meal of the day sets the mood for the rest of the day. Just as Larry felt better when he ate a breakfast of eggs and bacon most individuals with Reactive Hypoglycemic Tendencies are better regulated the rest of the day if they have fat and protein for breakfast. Still others with Reactive Hypoglycemic Tendencies do better if there is an emphasis on fat with a serving of fruit to start the day. For example, a smoothie made of cream and fruit with no added sugar can set the enteric brake "on" at the beginning of the day and influence the rest of the day compared to eating cereal for breakfast which can set the enteric brake "off" and influence the rest of the day detrimentally. It is important to eat soon after getting up so blood glucose doesn't drop while you are getting ready for the day. A bedtime snack containing some fat slows the absorption levels of glucose into the blood stream during the night which helps maintain adequate glucose levels throughout the sleeping time. The Zone Diet books may be helpful resources for menus and dietary suggestions.

The same vitamins, minerals and herbs can be helpful in reactive hypoglycemia regulation as are helpful in general hypoglycemia.

Specific suggestions given by patients include:

- Yams and asparagus are good to eat when I am having problems with my intestines shutting down. They seem to respond within

24 hours in a comfortable way not an explosive over response that I would get with other foods or medications I tried.

- Smoothies made of fruit and cream have helped me get the day started on the right foot. I have a blueberry/ strawberry/ raspberry with cream smoothie in the morning, about 6-8 ounces and then 3-4 ounces 2 hours later. My energy remains good and my blood glucose readings are stable and normal.

- Pizza made with white sauce, some meat and cheese other than American cheese along with a salad of veggies and greens provides a good dinner or lunch.

- At dinner I have chicken, fish or beef with veggies and a small portion of potato, rice or pasta. I fix a cream sauce using cream and butter to put over the protein and veggies, just a small amount is necessary. That can keep me stabilized for 2-4 hours depending how active I am in the evening.

- When I have a craving for sweets I have real ice cream, a choco-late, or butter cookie. These have a high ratio of fat to sugar so my gut tolerates the sugar a little better. I also eat the sweets after a meal so my gut is already set with good foods. Soft drinks, cakes and frosting, candy without fat will set my blood glucose dropping quickly and radically. My personality goes down the toilet too.

Exercise in moderation can help to stabilize blood glucose levels when done on a daily basis and at the same daily level of exertion. Exercise assists in balancing the body's hormonal levels in general and more specifically can be of benefit in maintaining level blood glucose because of a more stable insulin release by the pancreas and more stable glucose levels released by the gut.

Physiological Quieting has an important place in preventing reactive hypoglycemic symptoms. Stress increases hypoglycemic tendencies in fibromyalgia. Stress increases the levels of stress hormones such as cortisol and substance P. It decreases beneficial chemicals like the vitamin B complex, endorphins, and serotonin. If stress becomes a chronic way of life hormonal levels result in changes in insulin production and gut absorption.

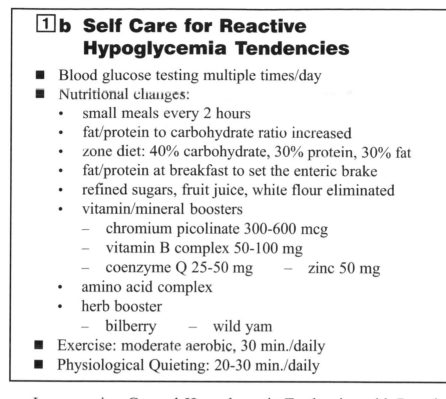

1 b Self Care for Reactive Hypoglycemia Tendencies

- Blood glucose testing multiple times/day
- Nutritional changes:
  - small meals every 2 hours
  - fat/protein to carbohydrate ratio increased
  - zone diet: 40% carbohydrate, 30% protein, 30% fat
  - fat/protein at breakfast to set the enteric brake
  - refined sugars, fruit juice, white flour eliminated
  - vitamin/mineral boosters
    - chromium picolinate 300-600 mcg
    - vitamin B complex 50-100 mg
    - coenzyme Q 25-50 mg   – zinc 50 mg
  - amino acid complex
  - herb booster
    - bilberry   – wild yam
- Exercise: moderate aerobic, 30 min./daily
- Physiological Quieting: 20-30 min./daily

In comparing General Hypoglycemic Tendencies with Reactive Hypoglycemic Tendencies it is noted that both cases exhibit imbalance between insulin and glucose in the bloodstream. In one case, that of General Hypoglycemic Tendencies, increased complex carbohydrate intake is a major factor in stimulating the appropriate insulin-glucose ratio in the bloodstream. In the other case, that of Reactive Hypoglycemic Tendencies, an increased protein and fat ratio to carbohydrates is a major factor in balancing the insulin-glucose ratio in the bloodstream. Each individual must use trial and error to determine his/her individual needs.

Amino Acid Necklaces

In some FMS individuals with hypoglycemic tendencies, using amino acid supplements with vitamin/mineral boosters has normalized the blood glucose readings and eliminated many of the symptoms. See Nutrition, Chapter 12.

Chapter 16

2 Hypothyroid Tendencies Self Stabilizing Loop

The Type 2 subcategory of fibromyalgia is termed hypothyroid tendencies.

Symptoms

Symptoms of hypothyroid tendencies include feeling cold, cold hands and feet, feeling core cold at times, weight gain, dry skin, heavy menstruation, PMS, and constipation. Additional complaints include fatigue, sleep disturbance, and stiff achiness rather than sharp pains. These descriptors may be from hypothyroid tendencies, a sluggish thyroid gland that is not producing adequate thyroid hormone or dysfunction of thyroid hormone at the cellular level. Thyroid hormone produced by the thyroid gland is an essential information molecule for many body functions. Another essential thyroid hormone is produced primarily at the cellular tissue level from hormone originating from the thyroid gland.

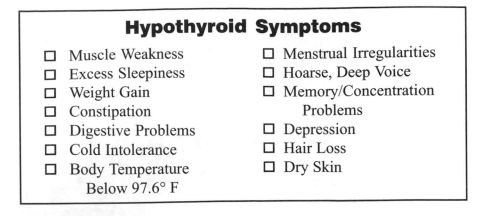

Hypothyroid Symptoms

- ☐ Muscle Weakness
- ☐ Excess Sleepiness
- ☐ Weight Gain
- ☐ Constipation
- ☐ Digestive Problems
- ☐ Cold Intolerance
- ☐ Body Temperature
  Below 97.6° F

- ☐ Menstrual Irregularities
- ☐ Hoarse, Deep Voice
- ☐ Memory/Concentration
  Problems
- ☐ Depression
- ☐ Hair Loss
- ☐ Dry Skin

Case Study

Margaret, a 35-year-old mother of three, complained to her health care professional about severe fatigue, overall stiffness and aching, headaches, PMS, weight gain, and a core feeling of cold. She began to crave chocolate bars and coke. Her thyroid function tests were normal but her basal body temperature was decreased. Her thyroid hormone T4 to T3 conversion was dysfunctional at the cellular level.

Etiology/Cause

Many times an individual with fibromyalgia complains of these "hypothyroid tendency" symptoms but the thyroid function test is normal. There is another form of thyroid chemical dysfunction that cannot be measured by blood tests. The symptoms have been documented in the medical literature since the 1970s. For our purposes this dysfunction will be termed cell level hypothyroidism.

Cell Level Problem

Cell level hypothyroidism is abnormal cellular T4 to T3 conversion. In other words the thyroid hormone T4 flows from the thyroid gland into the blood stream and then to magnet sites on body cells, for example to magnet sites on muscle cells. There T4 must be converted to T3 to be of use to the muscle cell in energy production. If that conversion does not take place, or is sluggish or incomplete, cell level hypothyroidism may result. Inadequate T3 at the cellular level can lead to stiffness, achiness, a decrease in basal body temperature, constipation and dry skin. T3 is essential for cell metabolism – lighting and maintaining the fire that produces energy in the cell. When the fire is hard to light, of low intensity, or erratic, outward symptoms appear.

An individual may have dysfunction at the thyroid level and at the cellular level simultaneously. In this case treating the thyroid level deficiency will alleviate some symptoms but the cellular level treatment will be necessary for more complete relief of symptoms.

Basic Physiology

To review thyroid function and its hormonal importance to body function we begin with the brain (Figure 16). The hypothalamus stimulates the pituitary gland in the brain which stimulates the thyroid gland in the neck region to produce T4 (Thyroxine). T4 is the foundation chemical needed to make the active thyroid chemical messenger T3 (Triiodothyronine).

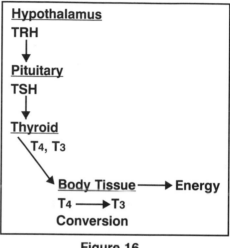

Figure 16

Approximately 80% of T3 formation occurs in the body cells not in the thyroid gland. T4 travels to the body cells via the blood stream so it can be measured in a blood test. T3 is produced in the tissue cells and remains there for the most part so a blood test does not indicate its level of production or effectiveness. T3 instructs body cells how fast or slow to operate and how hot the burners should be set to fire up the cellular activity. As such T3 is a major determinant of body temperature. A cell's burner is set high or low by T3. The test for T3 is Basal Body Temperature, the internal temperature of the body.

Metabolism and Temperature

Body temperature affects the overall metabolism of the body because the body's metabolism is the sum total of all the chemical reactions occurring in each cell. These chemical reactions are dependent on enzymes. Enzymes are the "sparks of life." There are digestive enzymes and metabolic enzymes. Think of chemical reactions in cells as the fire in each cell that provides the energy for the cell motor to run. Metabolic enzymes are the catalyst or stimulus that ignite the fire and helps determine the intensity of the fire that keeps the motor running. When temperature is decreased the enzymes are cold and stiff so the motor doesn't start easily, it sputters and runs only on one or two cylinders, quitting easily. When the temperature is increased, as when an individual has an illness with a high fever, the enzymes are too hot so the motor function (cell function) is abnormal to the point of destruction at times. When the temperature is decreased the cells go into a form of hibernation, when the temperature is increased greatly the cells burn up from an explosion of energy. The basal body temperature is designed to be 98.6°F, just the right temperature for the enzymes to act effectively and efficiently in the metabolic burn. In this state the cell motor can be active at a balanced steady state for long periods of time without fatigue, pain, or depletion of essential elements. The body is able to provide the nutrients the cell needs for its motor function and remove the waste products at a rate that is conducive to long term function. The individual feels warm, feels energetic, and feels pain free and alert. The skin is in a healthy state, the nervous system is healthy and the reproductive system is able to function in a healthy state.

We know that changes in body temperature change body functions. The body goes into a conservation mode when body temperature decreases. It ceases to provide energy production except where it is needed for vital organs. The skin becomes dry, hair becomes brittle and falls out, and the reproductive system becomes dysfunctional because these are not vital to minimal life. In the extreme, cells are destroyed and eventually organs die. Cell level hypothyroid tendency is experienced as a complex of symptoms brought on in part by alteration in body temperature.

Reproductive Hormones and Metabolism

The reproductive system affects thyroid function. Estrogen and progesterone facilitate thyroid function including the conversion of T4 to T3 at the cellular level. If estrogen/progesterone levels are decreased or the estrogen to progesterone ratio is abnormal there can be resultant changes in T4 to T3 conversion that will change the Basal Body Temperature and also result in cell level hypothyroid tendency symptoms.

ANS and Metabolism

The autonomic nervous system (ANS) significantly affects thyroid function. The enteric division determines the effective breakdown of protein, fat and carbohydrate nutrients to amino acids, fatty acids and sugars that the thyroid system can use in its synthesis and conversion of thyroid hormones. The sympathetic and parasympathetic divisions affect head brain function of the pituitary and hypothalamus glands that send messages to the thyroid. Both sympathetic and parasympathetic divisions send messages directly to the thyroid gland itself.

The Amino Acid Necklaces

The thyroid hormones are amino acid necklaces. The protein we eat is broken down in the intestines into 20-30 amino acids some of which combine to form the thyroid hormones T4 and T3. Protein contains approximately 16 percent nitrogen while the other basic nutrients, sugars and fatty acids, contain no nitrogen. Amino acid necklaces form the chemical messengers that transfer messages between nerve cells as well as facilitate the metabolism, the motor in each body cell. Lysine is an essential amino acid that aids in production of enzymes within the cell body as one of its functions. Tyrosine is an essential amino acid that is a precursor to norepinephrine the parasympathetic nervous system messenger. It is a vital ingredient in the function of the thyroid gland, the adrenal glands and the pituitary gland. Tyrosine attaches to iodine to form active thyroid hormones including T3. Symptoms of low tyrosine can include low body temperature, weight gain, low blood pressure, restless leg syndrome, depression and anxiety.

Blood Sugar and Metabolism

Blood sugar levels also affect cell level hypothyroid tendencies and body temperature. The reverse is also true. Low blood sugar or hypoglycemia, decreases body temperature and decreases metabolism. A diabetic with low blood sugar experiences cold sweats and uncontrolled shivering. High blood sugar levels increase the body's temperature and increases metabolism which can lead to hot sweats. Symptoms of hypoglycemia are very similar to cellular hypothyroidism.

HPA Axis and Metabolism

Cortisol levels also affect body temperature. Cortisol is produced by the adrenal glands and is part of the "stress" hormone package. High cortisol levels decrease body temperature and inhibit the conversion of T4 to T3 leading to cellular hypothyroidism. Use of cortisone can also lead to the same symptoms.

Test

The first assessment is a review of symptoms by the individual and a close family member or friend. (See Symptoms, page 154) A blood test can determine the level of thyroid hormone produced by the thyroid gland in an individual. The blood test does not indicate the level of T3 available at the cellular level because the great majority of T3 is converted from T4 at the site of metabolic activity.

To test for cell level hypothyroid tendencies use an oral thermometer and place it under your arm or in your mouth for 15 minutes while you remain quiet. If the temperature is 97.6° F or below, it can indicate an underactive T4 to T3 conversion level. Barnes recommended taking the temperature on awakening before getting up from bed. Wilson recommends taking it 3 times a day approximately 3 hours apart during the times of the day when symptoms usually occur. So if fatigue, pain, and coldness occur in the afternoon more than in the morning the tests would be predominately done from noon on.

Body temperature changes cyclically through the day in both sexes and through the month in females. It is usually lowest in the morning, highest in the afternoon and then decreases as the evening progresses. Additionally, for women, estrogen and progesterone, the information molecules from the ovaries cause variations in body temperature as they cycle during the month. Body temperature rises at ovulation (day 14) and just prior to the menstrual period. Temperature changes on the day of ovulation and three days before the menstrual period starts are not as accurate as during the rest of the month in diagnosing cell level hypothyroidism.

Treatment

Tyrosine and iodine are components necessary to form thyroxine, the thyroid hormone. If the amio acid tyrosine is low it may cause hypothyroid tendencies in FMS individuals Slagle describes using tyrosine and iodine to successfully treat hypothyroid tendencies.

Individuals with cell level hypothyroid tendency type symptoms may be helped by taking 2000-3000 mg Kelp daily for iodine and L-Tyrosine 500 mg 2 times daily for essential amino acid with water or juice, not with milk or other protein. For better absorption take the tyrosine with 50 mg B6 and 100 mg vitamin C. The tyrosine and iodine combine to form the active thyroid hormone T3.

Food sources of tyrosine include almonds, avocados, bananas, dairy products, lima beans, pumpkin seed and sesame seeds. Supplements of L tyrosine should be taken at bedtime or with a carbohydrate meal so it does not competing for absorption with other amino acids.

Adding phytoestrogen and/or progesterone in cream or food form may improve the symptoms of cell level hypothyroid tendency in individuals with fibromyalgia and reproductive hormonal dysfunction.

Fatty acids are also needed by the thyroid system to function effectively. Fatty acids are the building blocks of some messenger chemicals and come from the breakdown of fats and oils. Essential fatty acids (EFAs) cannot be produced in the body but must be supplied through the diet and broken down into fatty acid form in the gut. Fatty acids are needed for rebuilding and producing all cells in the body. Sources of essential fatty acids include fish oils, flaxseeds and flaxseed oil, grape seed oil and primrose oil. Amounts will vary depending on the supplement.

Vitamin B complex including Vitamin B12 is essential for cellular oxygenation and energy production. It is also needed for proper digestion of proteins into amino acids and fats into fatty acids. Fifty to 100 mg of vitamin B complex and 15-45 mg of vitamin B12 may be beneficial in facilitating cell metabolism and reducing "hypothyroid" symptoms.

The stomach digests apples and other fruits converting the fruit into malic acid along with other components. Malic acid is an essential acid for energy or ATP production at the cell level. Malic acid has the ability to increase utilization of needed substances including sugars for ATP production even under low oxygen conditions. It is a part of the efficient metabolism process in every body cell. Suggested malic acid intake is 1200-1400 mg/day.

The stomach and small intestine digests green leafy vegetables, legumes and nuts to obtain magnesium. Magnesium is the fourth most abundant mineral in the body. It is the number one stress mineral. ATP production is dependent on adequate magnesium levels at the cellular level. Magnesium facilitates enzyme function for metabolic action in each cell. It lights the spark (the enzyme) that lights the fire or starts the motor (metabolism) of each cell. It facilitates ATP energy into physical and mental function. Suggested magnesium intake is 500-800 mg/day.

Fluoride and chlorine are chemically related to iodine. These chemicals interfere with the body's ability to absorb iodine from food. They can block iodine receptors in the thyroid gland resulting in reduced iodine available in the thyroid and thus reduced iodine combined with tyrosine to form T4. Avoiding chlorinated water, fluoride toothpastes, and soy products may be of help in decreasing FMS symptoms.

Autonomic nervous system balance is necessary for optimal thyroid system function. Practicing Physiological Quieting on a daily basis can assist in balancing the system when it is in disequilibrium. These techniques include diaphragmatic breathing, hand warming and body-mind quieting.

Moderate aerobic exercise for 20-30 minutes daily facilitates hormonal, enzyme and nervous system balance. Walking, biking or swimming is recommended.

2 Self Care for Hypothyroid Tendencies

- Basal body temperature testing
- Nutritional changes:
  - kelp 1000-3000 mg
  - amino acids – L-tyrosine 1000 mg
  - vitamin B12 15-45 mg   • vitamin B6 50 mg
  - magnesium 400-600 mg   • essential fatty acids
  - avoid chlorine and fluoride
- Phytoestrogen and progesterone
- Exercise: moderate aerobic, 20-30 min/daily
- Physiological Quieting: 20-30 min/daily

③ Neurally Mediated Hypotension Self Stabilizing Loop

The Type 3 subcategory of fibromyalgia is termed neurally mediated hypotension.

Symptoms

Individuals with Neurally Mediated Hypotension Tendencies (NMH), also called vasomotor syncope, describe low blood pressure and high resting heart rate. Heart rate is often 90-100 beats per minute at rest when 60-70 is considered normal. Blood pressure is often 95/65 mm Hg when 110/70 is considered normal. These individuals describe feeling weak in the knees, dizzy and light headed, especially when getting up from lying or sitting. They describe mental and physical fatigue. Additionally they describe chest pain that so closely imitates heart problems a physician may do a complete cardiac workup, yet find nothing. They describe problems with swallowing and indigestion. They describe shortness of breath with minimal exertion. They describe abdominal pain that closely imitates pain from gall stones, interstitial cystitis, endometriosis, or canccr. As many as 60% of FMS individuals describe these symptoms.

Case Studies

Linda had six abdominal surgeries in three years to find what was causing the extreme pain and dysfunction. She had her gall bladder, loops of her intestine, her uterus, ovaries, and scar tissue removed. Nothing helped and she was worse after the surgeries at the end of three years. Clearly something else was producing the abdominal pain.

Melissa described her legs melting from under her while she was shopping. She felt her heart racing at times even when she was resting. She tired easily and quickly during her attempts at exercise or during recreational activities. She experienced such extreme discomfort and bloating in her abdomen that she could not wear clothing that touched her stomach. She had bouts of constipation and diarrhea. She burped unpleasant gas and experienced indigestion and stomach pain to a point that she was afraid to eat. Changing her diet did not help. Her abdominal pain increased before her menstrual cycle to the point she would often be in bed for several days with pain, weakness, nausea and vomiting. Her menstrual cycle was regular within 7-10 days. During her menstrual cycle the uterine cramping was intense. She described frequent feelings of urgency to toilet, getting up 1-2 times nightly and toileting every 1-2 hours. Yet, at other times Melissa felt great, energetic, athletic, and pain free.

Etiology/Cause

Neurally mediated hypotension is often overlooked as a possible cause for the symptoms of abnormal heart rate and blood pressure, chest and abdominal pain. The ANS-HPA-RHA messaging systems are not working together effectively to normalize heart rate, blood pressure, muscle and organ function in NMH. There is nothing wrong structurally with any of the organ systems. Rather it is the messaging systems that tell them what to do and how to do it that are dysfunctional. These dysfunctional messaging systems may also affect the blood flow to the organs which can lead to further symptoms at the organ level.

Melissa and others like her give us clues about how to help the symptoms. She told us, "When I feel terrible, if I go to McDonald's and have french fries I feel a lot better even though I know they are not good for me. My energy improves, my weak knees disappear, and my diarrhea improves."

Before we knew much about the heart and gut regulation centers and their potential affects on the rest of the body, Melissa's comments were baffling. To understand why McDonald's french fries helped Melissa and others with fibromyalgia it is necessary to understand some facts about the heart and gut control centers.

Gut Absorption and Heart Function

The body's serotonin, 95% of which is produced by the enteric nervous system of the gut, affects all cells of the body with receptor sites for serotonin. When the gut produces an abundance of serotonin it flows not only in the gut influencing the function there, but also to the brain, to the heart, to the blood vessels, to the uterus, and to the bladder. In the gut serotonin facilitates peristalsis, in the heart it increases the heart rate, in the blood vessels it stimulates constriction, in the uterus and bladder it induces contraction, and in the brain it facilitates sleep and decreases pain perception. Thus, the gut's enteric nervous system is an essential component in treating and controling fibromyalgia symptoms of high resting heart rate, low blood pressure and abdominal pain.

The gut's function is to digest food, absorb the digested nutrients into the blood stream and defend against poisons. The enteric nervous system controls the efficiency and effectiveness of these functions. It determines to a large extent what nutrients and how much of each nutrient are absorbed and how much are excreted in the feces/bowel movements. If salts from food are excreted in excess rather than being absorbed into the bloodstream, every cell of the body is affected in their ability to function optimally. Salts affect the dilation or constriction of blood vessels and the energy produced in muscle cells, just to mention two. A deficiency in sodium chloride salts results in blood vessel dilation, which results in the muscle we call the heart beating faster but less effectively, and in the skeletal muscles of the trunk, arms and legs contracting less effectively and relaxing incompletely. The human body can have a functionally low sodium chloride level that may or may not be detectable by the usual medical testing but the function of every cell of the body is affected by the lack of available salt. Increasing sodium chloride levels in the bloodstream so they are available to body cells will improve heart, blood vessel, and skeletal muscle function just to name a few.

Increasing sodium chloride in the diet of fibromyalgia individuals experiencing symptoms of high resting heart rate, low blood pressure, and abdominal pain may significantly improve the symptoms. When there is adequate sodium chloride, the blood vessels constrict/close more effectively which increases the pressure of the blood as it travels through them. Normal blood pressure results. The heart, in response to increased sodium chloride levels, slows the number of beats per minute and the pumping function becomes more effective and efficient. The skeletal muscles of the trunk, arms and legs are able to contract and relax quickly and completely in repetitive fashion when they have adequate sodium chloride. The muscle cells are thus able to receive the nutrients they need from the blood and lymph and can rid themselves of waste products effectively. Weakness, fatigue, pain, and stiffness decrease in the individual with fibromyalgia when there is adequate sodium chloride available to the cells.

Serotonin and Gut Pain

The enteric nervous system in FMS seems to oscillate between the extremes of activity or fatigue instead of holding to a middle ground of stimulating activity and rest. There is no balanced work-rest cycle. One example is the serotonin release by the enteric nervous system. Serotonin is released when there is pressure on the bowel lining cells. The serotonin excites peristalsis and thus elimination. If in the fibromyalgia gut the release of serotonin is excessive the peristalsis is initially increased which could cause diarrhea, dehydration and discomfort. As the serotonin continues to flow it "drowns" the magnet receptor sites in the gut and as with any drowning victim the sites cease to function so the gut shuts down. Excessive serotonin results in paralysis of the gut until the excess serotonin is broken down or otherwise incapacitated. Constipation and even impaction with inflammation results when the gut shuts down. Pain is present. Constipation and impaction of the gut is accompanied by abdominal pain, inability to stand up straight and a shuffling gait with quick fatigue. In severe cases, the individual cannot get up from a chair without help.

Improving the enteric nervous system function in the gut of fibromyalgia individuals experiencing symptoms of high resting heart rate, low blood pressure, and abdominal pain may significantly improve the symptoms.

When there is dysfunction or imbalance of the enteric system every other organ system in the body is potentially dysfunctional as well. The enteric nervous system communicates with the heart via the vagus nerve complex, it communicates with the pancreas which produces insulin via enteric peripheral nerves and information chemicals, it communicates with uterus and bladder much the same way. If the enteric nervous system is in a high activation mode the gut will transfer food from mouth to anus faster than usual. Additionally the uterus and the bladder can be more irritable, and the heart can beat faster. As a result, the muscles of the arms and legs receive oxygen and food products at a different rate and amount. The muscle cell metabolism is changed. Waste product removal is altered. The entire body is affected when the enteric nervous system of the gut is dysfunctional.

Testing

The diagnosis of NMH tendencies is most often based on a medical history, symptom diary and heart rate/blood pressure tests. If the symptoms are appropriate, the heart rate relatively elevated and/or the blood pressure low, NMH is considered as a subcategory type in FMS. There is a medical test to diagnose autonomic neurally mediated hypotension as this category is termed by some physicians. It is the tilt table test usually performed by a cardiologist. The individual is place on a tilt table, a table that has a foot rest and can be tilted from horizontal to vertical position in varying degrees. The table is tilted 70 degrees from horizontal for 45 minutes. The blood pools in the feet unless the heart works adequately and the veins in the legs and abdomen have adequate tone to push the blood back up to the heart and brain. When the autonomic nervous system is not responsive to the stress of the tilt the blood pressure drops and the heart rate does not increase adequately to keep the blood from pooling in the feet. The individual experiences widespread pain, fainting, nausea and even vomiting. Some individuals pass out. The sequelae may last several days after the test. Since the test is so aversive, it is not usually done until the individual tries a self care treatment approach and still has significant symptoms.

To determine if a food intolerance is part of the problem it is recommended that the individual eliminate that food product from the diet for 7-10 days and document any relief in symptoms. If the relief is significant then a change in diet is recommended.

Treatment

Initial treatment for NMH tendencies in FMS involves a self care routine. If the self care routine is not adequate then the tilt test is performed and specific medications can be prescribed.

Salt (NACL)

The first step in self care for NMH is to salt all foods, using salt during cooking, using bullion cubes in gravies and soups and taking salt tablets if exercising or perspiring alot. If that is not adequate to increase salt levels and decrease symptoms, the tests can be completed and medication prescribed.

Accentuate the Positive, Eliminate the Negative in the Enteric Nervous System (ENS)

The second step in self care for NMH is to assist the ENS in normal function. The ENS produces important chemical messengers that affect blood pressure and heart rate. These chemical messengers are formed from amino acid necklaces present in the gut so producing normal levels of these amino acid necklaces is important. Increasing protein and/or amino acid intake can be beneficial. A variety of meat and fish are needed because each contains different levels of the various amino acids. Another way to obtain the needed amino acids is through supplements containing amino acids with complementing vitamins and minerals.

Some food products stabilize and are beneficial to ENS production of chemical messengers that affect heart rate and blood pressure. Turkey contains high levels of tryptophan which is the precursor to serotonin so turkey will likely stimulate the ENS in a positive way. Milk products also contain tryptophan and can be useful in facilitating sleep and normalizing body functions. Applesauce, bananas, and rice have been known by every mother whose child has diarrhea to quiet the enteric system. When the ENS is sluggish, foods containing caffeine, spices like red pepper, and roughage can stimulate peristaltic action. Small amounts of these foods go a long way.

Sugars

Sugar (glucose) in the small intestine stimulates enteric nerve activity to gut and pancreas so insulin and glucose are released excessively. The result can be low blood sugar levels with symptoms being incoordination, weakness, confusion, agitation. The label is often given that this person has reactive hypoglycemia. See Chapter 15. Sugars ingested by a sugar sensitive individual with fibromyalgia would set off a cascade of events initiated by the enteric nervous system. Using the same rationale, eliminating simple sugars and presenting complex carbohydrates with fats and protein to the enteric nervous system could potentially prevent the hypersensitive reaction. The symptoms of fatigue, weakness, confusion, and personality change are significantly decreased or eliminated.

Fats

The fats taken into the digestive system slow the intestinal peristalsis. In the most drastic situation the enteric brake stops peristalsis all together until the fats are broken down by the bile salts into smaller molecules. Therefore fat intake can be used as an inhibitor of enteric nervous system activation of peristalsis. At the same time fat's quieting inhibitory effect on the enteric nervous system affects many other organ systems, i.e. bladder, uterus, heart, and has a quieting affect on them too.

Proteins

Proteins taken into the digestive system take longer for the enteric nervous system to break down than sugars and carbohydrates. The proteins tend to slow the enteric system's action. So a relatively high protein intake may help an individual with high resting heart rate and low blood pressure. The quieting affect of protein is not as great as the quieting affect of fat.

Eliminate Food Sensitivity

Eliminating food products that destabilize the ENS improves

chemical messenger production and function. Eliminate nicotine, caffeine and simple sugars. Hypersensitivity to certain foods can play a role in ENS dysfunction. When bloating, gas, alternating diarrhea and constipation is described food hypersensitivity may play a role in NMH tendencies. Lactose intolerance is the sensitivity to milk products. Wheat intolerance is the sensitivity to breads, pastas, and cereals containing any wheat. Even the thickening in gravies and stews or soups may contain wheat. Monosodium glutamate (MSG) intolerance is the sensitivity to an additive found in many prepared foods. The symptoms are very similar to NMH tendencies.

Dehydration

Dehydration is a major factor in gut dysfunction. It can cause constipation, fecal impaction and inflammation. Water in adequate amounts is a stimulus to gut peristalsis. Drinking 6-8 glasses of noncaffeinated fluid is the general recommendation. Individuals will state that they drink 6-8 glasses of fluid per day but if the majority of that is caffeinated or alcohol, both diuretics, the result is still dehydration.

Monitor Magnesium Levels

Individuals with low blood pressure need to monitor the amount of magnesium they take since magnesium is an effective smooth muscle relaxant. That means high levels of magnesium could potentially lower blood pressure even more. Since magnesium is low in some individuals with FMS there is a tendency to supplement at high levels. For the individual with FMS and low blood pressure, moderate levels of magnesium supplementation, 300-400 mg/day, is more often recommended. Blood pressure should be monitored when adding magnesium.

Alleviate Abdominal Discomfort

Individuals who experience abdominal discomfort with low blood pressure may have pelvic vein varicosities which result in pooling of blood in the lower abdomen. This can be especially pronounced in the week to 10 days before a period. It is no different than varicosities in the legs. Elevating the hips higher than the heart 2-3 times daily for 15-20 minutes and sleeping in a slightly head down position can facilitate drainage of these pelvic and uterine veins. Exercising in shoulder height warm water can pump the blood more efficiently from the legs and trunk to the heart because the water pressure is greatest at the deeper level, gradually decreasing the pressure from the legs and pelvis to the heart.

Use Essential Oils

The knowledge of essential oils is primitive in our western medical culture but in Chinese medicine they have been used for thousands of years. Essential oils of peppermint and chamomile have long been known to quiet the gut, i.e., the enteric nervous system. These can be taken internally in the form of teas. Essential oils can be applied externally over the abdominal or back area to relieve symptoms. They are combined with a carrier oil such as almond or olive oil. Example of oils that can be used externally include angelica, balm bergamot, clary, lavender, lemon verbena, mint, neroli, orange, and rose. Applying the oil daily with light massage over the abdomen and back has been of benefit.

Balance Heart Activity

The heart has its own intrinsic messaging system that to some extent controls its pumping action. The heart sends messages within itself and to other organ systems via electrical and chemical signals. The heart is the largest generator of electromagnetic energy in our body, far greater than the human brain. It responds directly to electromagnetic energy outside the body with electrical and chemical messages. The heart is the body's primary organizing force between the head and the body. The vagus nerve communicates between the head, heart and the gut.

Balancing the heart chemical and electrical messages can lower the resting heart rate and improve blood pressure. HeartMath, including the techniques of freeze-framing, cut-thru, and heart lock-in, teaches heart attention that helps the heart send a more balanced energy through the body. Moderate aerobic exercise, especially in warm shoulder height water can improve heart function and balance the heart brain messages.

Balance Breathing Activity

The breathing diaphragm is an integral part of the abdominal area and affects heart rate and blood pressure. Individuals with fibromyalgia exhibit dysfunctional breathing diaphragm patterns. The breathing diaphragm action decreases and/or becomes shallow and ineffective. It is unable to contract and relax effectively, at times remaining in a semicontracted, tight state for long periods. This can cause chest, abdominal and back pain since the breathing diaphragm attaches to the ribs, sternum (breast bone) and thoracic-lumbar spine. Accessory muscles of the neck and upper chest take over much of the breathing activity but breathing effectiveness and efficiency is compromised. The gentle movement of the internal organs with each breath is significantly decreased when accessory muscles take over the breathing pattern. Practice diaphragmatic breathing hourly for 30 seconds – just 4-5 breaths will do. Then practice longer periods of time before getting up in the morning and as you go to bed at night.

Diaphragmatic breathing practiced frequently throughout the day for short periods can improve many symptoms of fibromyalgia. Inhale let your belly button rise, exhale let your belly button fall. Quiet shoulders, quiet chest. Jaw released, tongue at the bottom of your mouth.

Balance ANS Activity

The heart, lungs, stomach, liver, pancreas, bladder, uterus, rectum and anus are all innervated and controlled by the autonomic nervous system – sympathetic and parasympathetic divisions. When there is pain and dysfunction in any of these organs the autonomic nervous system will be involved in a direct or indirect way. There is often a resulting imbalance between the parasympathetic and sympathetic input to organ function. Excitatory, survival messages to organs become more predominant and enduring rather than a balance of excitatory and quieting directions that allow the organs to work and rest in a healthy rhythm. This imbalance in autonomic nervous system messaging and the resultant organ response leads initially to superefficient organ function at high energy levels. But as with any machine or body system rest and maintenance is essential and in this picture there is little to no rest/maintenance cycle. The result is an eventual melt down of organ function with symptoms of pain, fatigue, indigestion, diarrhea, shortness of breath, and menstrual irregularity.

Returning a balance to the sympathetic-parasympathetic divisions of the autonomic nervous system is essential in improving symptoms of high resting heart rate, low blood pressure, chest and abdominal pain.

Physiological Quieting

Physiological Quieting is an effective and easy method of facilitating balance between the sympathetic and parasympathetic divisions. Using diaphragmatic breathing, hand warming, and body-mind quieting on a daily basis is recommended. Chapter 12 describes Physiological Quieting techniques.

Craniosacral Rhythm

Craniosacral rhythm is an effective method of facilitating sympathetic- parasympathetic balance. Any individual can learn the preliminary exercises while more complicated techniques are done by a trained clinician. With inhale rock your head back and your pelvis forward; with exhale rock your head forward and your pelvis back. The movements are small, slow and gentle. Combining this exercise with abdominal breathing gently balances the autonomic system by affecting the nerve roots as they exit the spine at the cranial and sacral areas for the parasympathetic system and at the thoracic and lumbar areas for the sympathetic system. These techniques also balance the flow of cerebral spinal fluid as it travels from the head brain down the spinal column and back up.

Balancing Exercise Activity

Exercise is difficult to do when your resting heart rate is over 90 beats/minute and your blood pressure is 95/60. The weakness, fatigue, and incoordination often keeps physical activity at a minimum. One of the best places to start exercising is in the pool. Shoulder height water provides over all body pressure greatest from the feet and gradually decreasing towards the shoulders. This pressure is a supplement to the body's own blood pressure to transfer the blood from the lower body to the heart. It enables you to exercise much longer without pain and exhaustion. Water also supports your arms and legs so exercise can be assisted or resisted by the water depending on how fast and vigorously you move.

At home, exercise in a reclined position initially. Then as your blood pressure and heart rate improve gradually do more exercise in the sitting and standing positions.

Use Physiological Quieting techniques to decrease your heart rate below 90 bpm before starting to exercise. Make sure that you are adequately hydrated before, during and after exercise.

▣ Self Care for Neurally Mediated Hypotension Tendencies

- Blood pressure and heart rate monitoring
- Nutritional changes:
  - salt, sodium chloride increase
  - magnesium levels monitored
  - caffeine, refined sugars, alcohol eliminated
  - amino acid complex increase
  - gut (enteric) normalizing foods
    - turkey, rice, applesauce, bananas
  - herb: licorice
- Pelvic vericosity drainage
  - hips higher than heart
- Essential oils
  - teas: peppermint, chamomile
  - external: angelica, balm, bergamot, clary, lavendar, mint, neroli
- Exercise: moderate aerobic, 30 min/daily
  - pool exercise with shoulder height water
- Physiological Quieting 20-30 min/daily

---

Chapter 18

4 Immune System Dysfunction Tendencies Self Stabilizing Loop

The Type 4 subcategory of fibromyalgia is termed immune system dysfunction tendencies.

Symptoms

Some individuals with fibromyalgia may experience immune system dysfunction that occurs in response to a chronic infection, sudden illness, surgery or medication use. The individual experiences mental and physical fatigue, sleep disturbance, muscle aching and weakness, and/or chronic flu or allergy like symptoms.

Etiology/Cause

The immune system is designed to prevent illness in general. More specifically the immune system is designed to prevent illness or dysfunction at an organ and cellular level. The immune system produces an army to defend against evil invaders. Defender molecules include white blood cells, antibodies, T cells and immunoglobulins. These defenders normally block attackers from attaching to body system cells. They prevent attackers from making an individual sick. When the immune system is weakened, the immune defenders are not able to block attackers that cause illness from attaching to magnet sites at the cellular level. When the attackers attach to magnet sites the organ system becomes "ill" with resulting body symptoms. This can cause additional infections, allergies, and organ dysfunctions. Since the immune system impacts every cell, every organ system, nervous system, and muscle system of the body, the impact of a weakened immune system is all encompassing. The weakened immune system may result in generalized "sick" symptoms and more specific symptoms in body systems that are most vulnerable. So in one individual the gut symptoms may be more dominant than the nasal symptoms or the lung symptoms. In another individual the musculoskeletal symptoms may be more dominant than heart, gut or lung symptoms. Fibromyalgia symptoms may often be influenced by the health of the immune system. If the immune system is weakened through genetic predisposition, through injury, yeast infection, nutritional deficiencies, environmental, chemical or mold sensitivities or other trauma, fibromyalgia like symptoms are often increased.

Candida/Yeast

Common yeast, Candida albicans, develops toxins which may weaken the immune system. The weakened immune system leads to additional toxin development. When yeast infections develop and spread through the mouth, throat, and intestines as well as the vaginal area, symptoms of diarrhea, constipation, abdominal pain, mental and physical fatigue, menstrual irregularities, and decreased body temperature may appear. Yeast infections often proliferate after use of antibiotics for other illnesses. The antibiotics kill the "bad" bacteria and so relieve the illness's symptoms. The antibiotics also kill the "good" bacteria that are naturally in the body. When the good bacteria are destroyed the remaining bacteria and other organisms can grow more rapidly and spread. Candida albicans is a fungus that is naturally present in limited amounts in the vaginal and gut tissues. Yeast is not harmed by antibiotics so these fungal cells grow in numbers and spread when other bacteria are killed by antibiotics.

Yeast growth may also increase when there is a high sugar intake. Sugar is food for yeast. The yeast fungal cells develop faster in a warm, sweet environment. When making bread, a combination of warm water, sugar and yeast produces gas and is used to give the bread lightness. Combining warm water, sugar and yeast in the body produces gas and proliferates yeast cells in the human body. Excessive yeast growth stimulated by sugar consumption may cause immune system dysfunction.

Testing

There is not a definitive medical test to determine yeast levels in the human body. Instead the diagnosis is often based on medical history and symptoms. The questions from the medical history that are important include:

- Have you been treated with antibiotics especially for a month or longer or four or more times in a twelve month period?
- Have you experienced problems in your reproductive organs i.e., vaginitis, urethritis, prostatitis for more than a month?
- Have you ever had fungal infections such as athlete's foot, nail or skin fungal infection that lasted more than a month?
- Do odors from perfume or insecticides cause symptoms that limit you from continuing normal activities?
- Do you crave sugar, bread, or alcoholic beverages?
- What symptoms do you have?

Crook lists the primary symptoms of yeast infection as fatigue, lethargy, poor memory, indecisiveness, numbness, burning or tingling, insomnia, muscle aches and weakness, abdominal pain, constipation and diarrhea, bloating, vaginal irritation and/or discharge, PMS, anxiety, and cold hands and feet.

Treatment

Treatment for yeast infections or symptoms from proliferation of yeast in an individual's body includes:

- Eliminating sugars to deprive the yeast of "food." Eating one or two fruits a day is still recommended. Drinking soda or fruit juice, eating candy, syrups, jellies or honey is not recommended.
- Adding acidophilus, a bacteria found in milk helps restore the bowel and gut to a healthy balance of yeast and bacteria. Yogurt is high in acidophilus so a cup of yogurt a day may be helpful. Acidophilus is also available in pill form.
- Adding carprylic acid/or garlic capsules and/or adding garlic to your cooking can restore gut balance and both may be natural alternatives to control yeast proliferation.

Nutritional Boosters

The immune system can also be weakened by nutritional deficiencies, environmental chemicals and molds, emotional stress, and viral infections. When nutritional deficiencies are a factor in immune system dysfunction dietary changes and the addition of nutritional supplements may be advisable. Coenzyme Q, also known as ubiquinone, is a nutritional supplement that may stimulate immune system function, and decrease fatigue and blood pressure according to medical research. Vitamin B12 supplements have been shown to decrease fatigue in the absence of anemia in a double blind study by Ellis. Nutritional supplements, especially vitamin B12 and Vitamins C and E, improve immune system function. The HPA axis and immune system function can be facilitated using nonprescriptive herbs including Licorice, Panax Ginseng, Echincea and Vitamin C. Essential fatty acids are another supplement that may be beneficial for immune system related fibromyalgia symptoms. Omega 6 essential fatty acids are found in some fish oils, flax oil and evening primrose oil. Improvement in dizziness, depression, memory loss, and mental and physical fatigue have been noted. Echinacea is an herb which can stimulate the immune system. It can improve the defense system of the individual with fibromyalgia. Goldenseal is another herb that stimulates the immune system. Use of these herbs should be limited to 2-3 weeks at a time since the immune system could become overstimulated and then fatigued again. The idea is to find a balance for the immune system activity so it can effectively maintain the body's health.

Environmental Chemicals

There are chemicals and molds that are toxic to most individuals coming in contact with them. Some individuals with fibromyalgia experience severe chemical and mold sensitivity to the point that most chemicals and molds must be kept away from the individual. In these instances the individual's home and work environment must be as dust free, chemical free, and mold free as possible. Carpets are removed and walls and floors are disinfected with natural cleaners, chemicals used in cleaning are removed, chemicals used in cooking are eliminated.

Physiological Quieting

Emotional stress has an impact on immune system function. Emotional stress activates the HPA (Stress) axis, increasing cortisol and norepinephrine levels which stimulate the immune system. There is an initial boost in immune system response to the stress event. If the stress becomes chronic in nature the HPA axis and the immune system "fatigue" acting more erratically and then becoming exhausted.

Physiological Quieting (PQ) decreases the impact of emotional stress on the HPA axis and the immune system by refocusing the body's responses to efficiency of all organ and body systems within a short time. Physiological Quieting prevents the stress response from becoming ongoing and fatiguing the immune system. Physiological Quieting impacts the immune system more directly via its organ components, i.e. the pituitary, hypothalamus and adrenal glands and their hormone production. PQ facilitates these organs in a balanced approach to hormone production and work rest cycles.

Exercise

Exercise in moderation stimulates the immune system balance. The key is moderation, since too much exercise can stress the immune system causing an increase rather than a decrease in symptoms. Twenty to 30 minutes of moderate exercise is a goal to strive for. It is possible that the individual may need to start at 3-5 minutes initially and gradually increase the length of time.

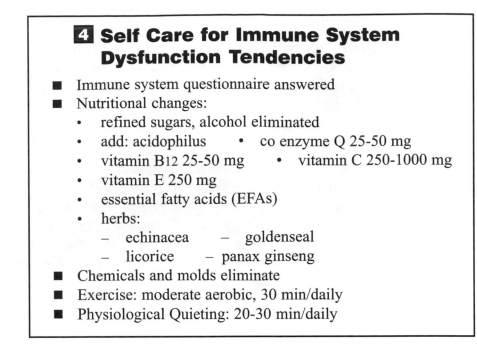

4 Self Care for Immune System Dysfunction Tendencies

- Immune system questionnaire answered
- Nutritional changes:
  - refined sugars, alcohol eliminated
  - add: acidophilus   • co enzyme Q 25-50 mg
  - vitamin B12 25-50 mg   • vitamin C 250-1000 mg
  - vitamin E 250 mg
  - essential fatty acids (EFAs)
  - herbs:
    - echinacea   – goldenseal
    - licorice   – panax ginseng
- Chemicals and molds eliminate
- Exercise: moderate aerobic, 30 min/daily
- Physiological Quieting: 20-30 min/daily

Chapter 19

5 Reproductive Hormonal Imbalance Self Stabilizing Loop

The Type 5 subcategory of fibromyalgia is termed reproductive horomonal imbalance tendencies.

Symptoms

These individuals describe monthly and/or yearly cycles of increased muscle pain, fatigue, sleep disturbance, menstrual irregularities, bowel and bladder irritability and depression.

Case Studies

Mary experienced incapacitating symptoms of body pain, fatigue, abdominal bloating, and gut dysfunction by Thanksgiving every year. She would miss work and school and would be in bed much of the time. She felt weak and fatigued. Mentally she was depressed and when she tried to work she found she made many mistakes. She would try medications and food elimination without help. Using phytoestrogen and progesterone creams she was able to return to work and attend school. She did not become ill or need to limit her activities any more than other times of the year. She states she has confidence that her life is under more control and balance.

Joann described extreme symptoms the week before her menstrual cycle. She experienced fatigue, muscle pain, shakiness, and sleep disturbance. The abdominal pain at the beginning of menstruation incapacitated her for 1-3 days. She began using flax seed in her smoothie each morning and used phytoestrogen during the first 14 days of her cycle.and progesterone during the end of the month. Her menstrual cycle became more regular and the pain and fatigue along with the sleep disturbance improved to the point she was not missing work or school. She described her energy level and optimism improving to the point she would plan trips away from home during the week before her menstrual cycle was to begin.

Cause/Etiology

Estrogen and progesterone hormones (chemical messengers) produced primarily in the ovaries affect all organ systems including the head, the gut, and the muscles. They are produced from essential fatty acids and cholesterol. Estrogen facilitates the build up of edometrium in the uterus. It tends to increase blood pressure. Additionally estrogen facilitates sleep, a sense of well being, increased energy, increased endorphins (the natural body endorphins), and increased serotonin. It facilitates absorption of calcium through the intestine and increases blood flow to the brain and muscles. It facilitates thyroid hormone conversion of T4 to T3. Progesterone facilitates slowing of the digestive system and tranquilizing mood, it increases appetite, sex drive, and water retention in the body, facilitates breast engorgement and decreases blood pressure. (Figure 17)

Estrogen	Progesterone
Increases Blood Pressure	Decreases Blood Pressure
Increases Sleep	Decreases Digestive Activity
Inceases Well Being	Increases Appetite
Increases Energy	Increases Sex Drive
Increases Endorphins	Increases Water Retention
Increases Seratonin	Increases Breast Engorgement
Increases Calcium Absorbtion	Decreases Feeling of
Increases Brain Blood Flow	Well Being
Increases Muscle Blood Flow	
Increases Thyroid Function	

Figure 17: Impact of Estrogen and Progesterone

Estrogen and progesterone vary on a monthly (28 day) cycle in the female. Estrogen rises more than progesterone during the first 14 days of the cycle. At ovulation (day 14) estrogen and progesterone. After ovulation, progesterone rises more than estrogen for the last 14 days. Then both decline with the initiation of the menses (period).

Reproductive hormones influence the circuitry in the central nervous system and the way the brain processes information. Hormonal changes that occur during the menstrual cycle can have profound effects on the way information is integrated in the central and peripheral nervous system. In one study testing ischemic pain (pain from lack of blood circulation), women expressed increased pain levels during the last 14 days of the menstrual cycle compared to the first 14 days. The last 14 days of the menstrual cycle is associated with higher levels of estrogen, progesterone and lutenizing hormones (female hormones). The masculinizing hormones (like testosterone) are minimized in their effect during this time. Male hormones minimize pain perception compared to female hormones which accentuate pain perception. Opiods are important in regulating the menstrual cycle and ovulation so pain exacerbation in FMS individuals during the last 14 days of the menstrual cycle may be related to the fact that opiod levels that are decreasing.

Estrogen/progesterone levels can affect muscle strength. Some females lose as much as 9-10% of muscle strength during the week before the menstrual period starts.

Estrogen and progesterone varies on a yearly cycle too. Estrogen and progesterone fall in the winter and rise in the summer. The transition times are fall and spring. Estrogen and progesterone will be at their highest level during April through July and at their lowest from October through January. This may help to explain the reports of increased FMS symptoms during the winter months. When individuals complain of increased symptoms during the winter months it may be that the estrogen/progesterone levels have fallen excessively much like the occurrence at the end of the monthly cycle. If increased symptoms occur in the spring it may be an over abundance of estrogen/progesterone or a ratio variation between estrogen/progesterone and testosterone.

In one study progesterone levels were found not to change throughout the month in FMS individuals. There was a significantly higher incidence of galactorrhea (milky discharge of breasts), polycystic ovaries, endometriosis, uterine fibroids, and ovarian cysts. This imbalance may result in higher than normal levels of progesterone in relation to estrogen during the first part of the cycle and lower than normal progesterone in relation to estrogen levels the second 14 days. This imbalance could cause chronic immune system activation and eventually immune system fatigue and dysfunction.

When the ratio of estrogen to progesterone is abnormal the potential for sleep disturbance, fatigue, muscle pain, depression and confusion can increase. As estrogen decreases calcium absorption drops leading to muscle pain and fatigue. Thyroid hormone T4 conversion rate to T3 decreases. This leads to metabolism abnormalities at the cellular level. Fatigue, sluggishness, hunger, and feeling cold are symptoms of dysfunctional metabolism. Decreased circulation to the brain and decreased potentiation of serotonin and enkephalins in the brain can lead to mental confusion, depression, and memory problems.

The ratio of estrogen/progesterone to testosterone levels are another consideration in FMS symptoms. Testosterone, the male hormone, facilitates muscle definition and strength and the distribution of fat around the waistline but also decreases pain perception. An imbalance in the ratio of estrogen/progesterone to testosterone can aggravate muscle spasms and increase pain perception.

Relaxin

Relaxin is a little known hormone present in both females and males that may also affect fibromyalgia symptoms. Relaxin is produced in the ovaries, uterus, and breast tissue in the female. In the male it is produced in the seminal tubule. Relaxin levels vary throughout the month in females in conjunction with the estrogen-progesterone cycle. It is usually measurable in the blood stream seven to ten days after ovulation in females. It is difficult to measure in males. During pregnancy relaxin is present at levels ten times higher than in the non-pregnant state. It is the third major pregnancy hormone, estrogen and progesterone being the other two. Relaxin affects the production, elasticity and remodeling of collagen which is a major component in muscle, ligaments and tendons. Relaxin, through its affects on collagen synthesis and remodeling, causes ligaments and connective tissues to elongate and relax. It also affects the smooth muscle tone of blood vessels, increasing dilation of vessels at peripheral sites. Relaxin receptor sites have been found in brain tissue, smooth muscle of the gut and heart, and connective tissue including hair follicles and skin. Women who are perimenopausal, postmenopausal, have had a hysterectomy, oophorectomy, tubal ligation, or extended use of birth control pills which suppress ovarian functions have had the source of relaxin critically diminished. These same women may be at higher risk for fibromyalgia symptoms.

FMS individuals often report a significant decrease in symptoms during pregnancy and while they are nursing. The rise in relaxin levels may be involved in this dramatic change for these women. It is postulated that FMS individuals have a systemic deficit in making and/or utilizing the hormone relaxin. This leads to stiffness, pain, decreased circulation, and sleep disturbance.

Oxytocin

Oxytocin is another female hormone found to often be imbalanced in FMS individuals. Oxytocin is a regulator of the autonomic nervous system and blood pressure. Oxytocin regulates blood circulation in small diameter vessels i.e., in hands and feet and smooth muscles. As such it can be a factor in neurally mediated hypotension. It assists the brain in concentration. Oxytocin improves sex drive. It is part of the regulatory mechanism of the gastrointestinal tract. In several studies it has been shown to have an analgesic effect throughout the body. Oxytocin is also produced in the retina of the eye so decreased levels can cause vision problems. It is produced in the pineal gland, the same gland that produces melatonin, the sleep enhancing hormone. Oxytocin facilitates deep sleep levels possibly by facilitating melatonin's effect. Oxytocin production in the brain and the enteric nervous system may relieve anxiety and fear. Some physicians recommend oxytocin 5-10 units/day along with DHEA and T3 thyroid hormone, malic acid, magnesium, choline and inositol.

DHEA

Dehydroepiandrosterone (DHEA) is a steroid hormone, a weak cousin of testosterone that is needed for cellular growth and repair. It is an immune system booster. It is a controlling factor in skin oil and hair growth so excess DHEA can lead to acne and increased facial hair. In FMS individuals DHEA is often lower than normal (129 vs 192). J. Teitelbaum reports suboptimal levels of DHEA in FMS individuals 70-80% of the time. He recommends blood levels for men be 350-480 mg/dl and women be 150-180 mg/dl. J. Flechas recommends 25-50 mg at bedtime to improve DHEA levels. Prescription doses are often better quality but DHEA is available over the counter. DHEA is considered the single best neurochemical indicator for stress levels in the body by some medical professionals.

Test

The test for hormonal levels of estrogen and progesterone is available through a home spit test. This test measures the estrogen/progesterone levels at one point in time. The daily diary of symptoms can provide information about the cyclical nature of the symptoms over a months time.

Treatment

Supplementing with phytoestrogens and/or progesterones in food or cream form or using hormone replacement therapy on a temporary or permanent basis may assist the organ systems in balanced function. Self care treatment can include using phytoestrogen and phytoprogesterone on a cyclical basis. Over the counter creams can be used. Phytoestrogens are available in foods such as soy, flax seed, and green tea. Many vegetables have natural estrogen components- green beans, carrots, peas, and beets are a few. Fruits have estrogen components too – they include cherries, apples and rhubarb. Phytoprogesterones are in soybeans and yams. Prescription hormone replacement therapy is also available. In a clinical trial, pain and fatigue, bowel, bladder and menstrual cycle dysfunction improved in a small group of women who used phytoestrogen and progesterone during the winter months and again in the spring.

Relaxin is available in nonprescription form as a nutritional supplement.

Oxytocin is available in prescription form only.

DHEA is available in prescription or nonprescription forms. It also can be restored and maintained by joy, sexual activity, physical exercise, positive thinking and sunshine. Vitamin C (2000 mg/day) and Methyl Sulfonyl Methane (1000 mg/day) may be of benefit in raising the DHEA levels. Yams, used in manufacturing DHEA, cannot be used by the body to convert to DHEA. Shealy has found topical progesterone cream (UPS grade 3%), 1/4 teaspoon twice daily has sometimes facilitated increased DHEA levels. In a study by Meely adding 50mg of DHEA daily improved reproductive hormone levels, skin integrity, energy levels and mood stability.

---

5 Self Care for Reproductive Hormone Dysfunction Tendencies

- Hormonal tests and monthly symptom diary
- Nutritional changes:
  - estrogen/progesterone rich foods
    - soy, flax seed, green tea
  - caffeine, refined sugars eliminated
  - vitamin C 250-1000 mg
- Nonprescriptive creams or supplements:
  - phytoestrogen cream   – phytoprogesterone cream
  - DHEA
  - phytoestrogen/progesterone supplements
- Fun, laughter, joy
- Exercise: moderate aerobic, 30 min/daily
- Physiological Quieting: 20-30 min/daily

Chapter 20

What Can I Do
To Stay Physically Fit?

Joyce Dougan, P.T.
Barbara Penner, P.T.
Janet A. Hulme, P. T.

Physical fitness develops through regular exercise, 20 to 30 minutes daily as a maintenance dose. It becomes part of a routine like brushing your teeth or combing your hair. It may seem like an effort at first but eventually the individual with FMS does not want to miss it.

Start an exercise program with just a few activities and a few repetitions (three to five), then progress as tolerated. Be the tortoise and not the hare. It is better to successfully get to the finish line than start fast and burn out. Try to do a few activities several times a day rather than doing a lot at one time once a day. The more frequent exercise/stretches help keep the FMS individual from getting so sore and stiff throughout the day. It is also a good way to breakup sustained activities such as typing, sitting in class, driving, or standing.

Start out your morning with "stretch and yawn" while still in bed. This is doing what feels good, not a specific set of stretches. This is what small children do when they awaken . . . be a kid again! Doing neck and upper back stretches works especially well in a hot shower. (Figure 18) Then doing positional bed exercises for several minutes each can be beneficial (Figure 19). Doing shoulder shrugs and rolls, performing head rolls side to side, stretching arms forward and back, are simple activities that can be done seated or standing as a work break. They can be completed in less than a minute so work flow is not interrupted. In fact, the mini exercise routine will likely increase the individual's concentration and productivity.

A few stretches or exercises at lunch and coffee breaks help relax the muscles that have been used during work and increase blood flow to the area while decreasing tension. Another good time for the FMS individuals to take a few minutes for him/herself is after work and before tackling the evening activities. Even 15-20 minutes between work and dinner to recline using positional stretches can help. When not working outside the home, it is important to develop a daily routine. In addition to bed and shower stretches, doing some stretches and exercises after breakfast, mid morning, after lunch and before dinner helps with pain and stiffness. Another approach is to set a timer and do exercises every two hours for 3-5 minutes.

Posture

Standing and sitting posture is the base from which movement occurs. In FMS during standing it is common to see forward head, elevated, rounded shoulders, knees as straight as possible and locked with the weight pressing back, and weight acceptance on one leg more than another. The shoulder and neck muscles are over active and seem to hold the body up. The head and shoulders often lead during walking.

It is important to understand that standing posture should be maintained primarily by the bony skeleton and ligaments, not muscle action. There is minimal activity of the ankle muscles to maintain balance but the shoulder muscles, the abdominal and buttocks muscles should be relaxed. To stand in the most effective pain-free posture:

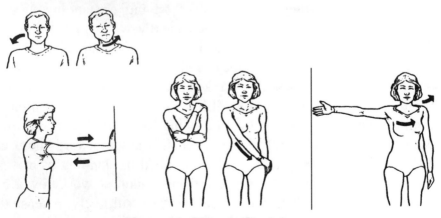

Figure 18: Shower Stretches

- Take weight equally on both feet.
- Unlock both knees.
- Push the top back of the head towards the clouds. Let the chin drop slightly as the spine lengthens.
- Release shoulders, thinking of the shoulder and neck muscles as a velvet cloak resting on a hanger (the skeleton).
- Release jaw, teeth apart, tongue released from the roof of the mouth.
- Slow, low diaphragmatic breath in the low abdomen.

Once the standing posture is comfortable, progress to:

- Weight shift in small amplitudes side to side.
- Perform slow, small knee bends.
- Weight shift front to back with one foot in front of the other.

During these exercises, lead with the hips, keeping the shoulders and neck released and relaxed. Maintain slow, low diaphragmatic breathing.

To sit in the most effective, pain-free posture:

- Take weight equally on both feet.
- Take weight equally on both hips.
- Push the top back of the head towards the clouds. Let the chin drop slightly as the spine lengthens.
- Release shoulders, thinking of the shoulder and neck muscles as a velvet cloak resting on a hanger (the skeleton).
- Release jaw, teeth apart, tongue released from the roof of the mouth.
- Slow, low diaphragmatic breath in low abdomen.

Once the sitting posture is comfortable, progress to the following exercises:

- Weight shift from side to side, one hip to the other. Increase the distance between ribs and hip on the side taking the weight.
- Weight shift front to back, rock the pelvis front to back over the thighs.

During these exercises, lead with the hips, keeping the shoulders and neck released and relaxed. Maintain slow diaphragmatic breathing.

Stretching

The goal of stretching is to increase the ease of pain-free movement. For the individual with FMS the technique for stretching a tight muscle is different than a "feel good" full motion stretch. Stretching needs to be done when the body is warm and relaxed. This can be accomplished in a hot shower, after a warm bath, after 5-10 minutes of heat application, or following active exercise. Muscles need to be stretched slowly just until the beginning of discomfort is noted, concentrating on avoiding pain. Breathe into the stretch for 15-30 seconds. Think slow, small, soft, smooth, sensitive stretch. The breath is low, use diaphragmatic breathing. Stretching to "pull out" the tightness doesn't work. It can set off more muscle tightening. Return to neutral slowly and smoothly to avoid rebound tightening. One to three repetitions is enough. The typical stretch to the end of range with overpressure sets off the already overactive stretch reflex and feeds into the high resting tone (gamma bias) present in FMS muscles. Figure 18 shows appropriate shower stretches.

The goals of stretching can be accomplished through positional stretches. Positional stretches are each held for 3-5 minutes while resting on a mat or bed. (Figure 19)

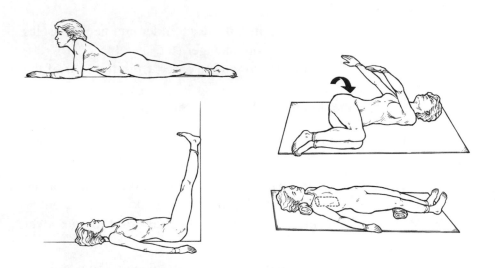

Figure 19: Positional Stretches

Strengthening

If the word strengthening brings to mind visions of Arnold Swartzenegger, don't be overwhelmed. The goal is not to be bursting with muscles, but to have enough strength to complete daily tasks and an extra reserve to allow more than the bare necessities. Strengthening may need to begin with using the weight of the FMS individual's own arm or leg as the weight. The starting point may be to move the arm as high as the shoulder 3-5 times and only gradually increase the height of the lift until it can move overhead without pain. Leg strengthening might begin with standing at the kitchen counter and rolling up and down from heels to toes or lifting a leg out to the side. Move through the exercises like floating on a cloud. Alternate movement with relax/release. Rest periods are important between each movement. Maintain a regular breathing rhythm without breath holding during the exercise. Avoid repetitively slowly lowering arms and legs from a raised position – this is called an eccentric contraction – and is more fatiguing than moving them up and down.

Once exercise endurance has increased to ten repetitions of any one exercise without fatigue or residual soreness, weight or resistance can be used. Since commercial weights start at one pound it may be better to start with a 4-6 oz. can of tuna or mushrooms. Progress to 8 oz. of tomato paste, then 10 oz. of soup. Progress through the cupboard until a one pound weight is tolerated. If gripping a weight increases forearm pain, put dried beans or popcorn (unpopped, of course!) in a zip lock bag or in a knee high nylon and tie it around the wrist. It should slide on and off and allow the hand and forearm muscles to remain relaxed. Sometimes weights cause increased pain during and after exercise. This may be due to the resistance during the slow lowering portion of the exercise, the resistance while returning to the rest position. Elastic bands or tubing is recommended as an alternative since there is no additional resistance during the eccentric portion of the exercise.

Large elastic bands or tubing come in a range of resistance from easy to difficult. The amount of resistance can be varied within one band by shortening it to make it harder or lengthening it to make it easier to pull against. A variety of exercises can be done with one band with a minimum of effort, whereas a series of weights are needed for different exercises. In FMS, elastic bands sometimes enable more exercise repetitions without soreness when compared to weights.

Aerobic Exercise

Aerobic exercise is designed to deliver oxygen to tissues efficiently and improve heart and lung function. An individual with FMS needs to perform moderate aerobic exercise 5-6 times a week. Initially ask, "What can I do without increased pain?" Begin with "soft" non weight bearing exercises such as bicycling or water aerobics. Resting heart rate before starting exercise needs to be under 100 beats per minute, preferably 55-65 beats per minute. Use Physiological Quieting before aerobic exercise to lower heart rate and release tight muscle areas.

For inactive FMS individuals experiencing pain, start with a two minute warm up of gentle stretches with breathing, then perform three minutes of moderate exercise that increases heart rate towards the target heart rate. Then perform two minutes of warm down stretches with breathing release. Pool exercises in warm water (85°F) at shoulder height enables more movement without pain.

For active FMS individuals already exercising but still experiencing pain, start with a 5-10 minute warm up of stretches, then progress to moderate exercise so there is not significant pain during or at the completion of the exercise. Insert rest cycles between shorter exercise cycles. For example, an individual may be used to running three miles daily, feeling pain increase after two miles and being exhausted and painful for 4-6 hours after completion of the workout. The modified workout after warm up stretches would be running one mile, resting and/or walking for five minutes, running for one mile, resting and/or walking for five minutes, then running for one mile, and cool down. If the individual is still sore and fatigued for 4-6 hours, decrease the work sets to one-half to three quarters of a mile each. End the exercise period with 5-10 minutes of cool down stretches. Doing the post exercise stretches and relaxation in a hot tub or under a hot shower is advisable to increase circulation that has decreased abnormally in the FMS individual's muscles.

Since FMS individuals' breathing patterns become erratic during exercise, it is important to be conscious of diaphragmatic breathing during aerobic exercise and rest cycles. Start with exercise that enables the maintenance of comfortable, rhythmical breathing. Some individuals will begin with walking a few blocks, a few lengths of a hallway or keeping time or dancing to one song on the radio. Aerobic activity utilizing equipment includes using a bike, treadmill, cross country ski machine, or steps. FMS individuals are often prone to hypoglycemia during and after exercise. To prevent hypoglycemia during exercise it is recommended that a small carbohydrate snack is eaten immediately before exercise and a larger carbohydrate/protein meal is eaten within 30 minutes after exercise. In addition it is important to prevent dehydration during exercise by drinking 6-8 oz. of water every 30 minutes during exercise.

Improvement in aerobic conditioning can be expected in 12-20 weeks, not in the six weeks expected aerobic progression with a non-FMS individual. The most important considerations are consistency of exercise and gradual increase in exercise tolerance. It is common to reach plateaus that last weeks or even a month or two. Don't give up. Maintain the exercise level that is comfortable.

When joining a group activity or joining a friend for tennis, golf, or bowling, the FMS individual may need to modify some of the movements or the pace to allow work within his/her limits. Start with fewer games or holes then gradually work up .

When starting with a new exercise or weight, do only 3-5 repetitions and see if there is any soreness the next day. Do not do a lot the first time even though there isn't any feeling of discomfort because the soreness may be delayed for several hours or even a day. If the same level of exercise is tolerated for three to four days without any negative effects then it is permissible to increase weight or repetitions, but only increase one of these at a time. Increase 1-2 repetitions at a time. Increase by a quarter to one half pound at a time. Give the 3-5 repetition prescription to any physical therapist that helps you.

Pool Exercises

Most exercises can be accomplished with less pain and faster progression if done in a warm pool. Aerobic exercise is also very effective in shoulder level warm water. The recommended target heart rate is approximately 20% less than recommended target heart rate for aerobic exercise on land. Aerobic endurance improves from 3-5 minutes for the acutely painful FMS individual to 45 minutes with 1-2 rest periods when the pain and fatigue has decreased. There should be no pain during pool exercise. The FMS individual should feel better at the end of the session even though there is a tired feeling. It is common for an individual to comment that it seems so easy in the pool. It is important not to overdo initially. Build up gradually. Always keep warm, using a hot tub or sauna and warm shower before and after the exercises. The pool temperature is best between 87-92° F to increase circulation and improve muscle relaxation. Being shoulder height in water eliminates 80% of gravity's pull on the body so movement can be the most efficient and pain-free.

Warm Up Stretches

(Don't forget to breathe.)
- Neck – forward/back to neutral, side bend, rotation
- Shoulders – hand to opposite shoulder
- Wrist – forward/back, circles each direction, turn palms up/down
- Leg/hip – hamstring stretch, Achilles stretch, roll knees out and in

Exercises in Standing

- Standing arm exercises while marching
  - Arms forward/backward
  - Hand circles
  - Hands to opposite shoulders
  - Arms forward & back - hand to face height
  - One hand on abdomen, one hand on low back, then reverse
  - Elbows to shoulder height, then down
  - Bend elbows, push down

- ■ Standing leg exercises
  - • Marching
  - • Weight shift side to side, feet apart
  - • Rock forward (elbows back), rock back (arms forward)
  - • Leg out to side
  - • Leg back & forward
  - • Leg circles

- ■ Arm and leg exercises
  - • Hand to opposite knee
  - • Hand toward opposite foot
  - • Hand to inside heel
  - • Hand to outside heel
  - • Hands to right, legs to left – twist, then reverse

■ Water walking - forward, backward, side crossovers

Chapter 21

What Can I Do To Stay Emotionally Healthy?

Ellen S. Silverglat, M.S.W
Janet A. Hulme, P.T.

Having an illness lets us know that an individual is not invulnerable to the problems that others suffer. People like to believe that illness and accidents happen to others. Sometimes an FMS individual resorts to superstition to reassure him/herself. As a part of an audience at a presentation where the odds of getting a disease or having an accident are stated, think about the fact that people all through the group are counting friends and family who have already had the problem and then giving a sigh of relief as if some quota had been met that spared them. It is easy to spot unrealistic perceptions of invulnerability or even immortality among adolescents. Adults are less obvious but it lingers on in many people. To admit that you can develop a medical problem is to admit lack of control and the absence of guarantees in our lives. Often people ask, "Why has this happened to me?" which almost sounds like others deserve the problem. Acknowledging that unwanted changes can happen may affect our self image if it was believed previously that illness equals weakness or lack of sufficient vigilance on our part to stay well. Just as an individual is not wholly defined by his/her work, his lineage, his physical attributes or any other single factor, he/she is not defined by this state of health. Part of the work of staying emotionally healthy is remembering how complex each individual is. Reduced strength in some areas doesn't cancel an individual's personality. Modification of how an individual performs daily activities doesn't cancel wit, sense of humor or other good or bad traits.

Accurate Information

An individual's opinions of him/herself may be based on inaccurate information and lead to harsh self appraisal. Information about what each individual must deal with can alleviate a lot of self blame, feelings of persecution or disappointment resulting from unrealistic expectations. Although the fund of information on fibromyalgia may be incomplete, it is a healthy thing to seek reliable information. Being well informed is part of being a responsible person. The unknown is often worse than reality and fear of the unknown leads to increased anxiety and poor coping. Watch out for myths such as "all illnesses are acute, lab tests and x-ray can diagnose everything, there are cures for almost everything, strength of will can overcome any disease" or the devastating thought that "chronic illness means a meaningful life is ended." Positive thoughts alone may not be a cure but they can greatly enhance coping. Negative thoughts can make any illness worse and immobilize coping abilities.

Active Participation

What does it mean that an FMS individual has a need to see one or more health care professionals? It doesn't mean he/she must or should relinquish all decision making to these people. Sometimes it is hard to remember that the individual is a very important part of his/her care. Many times an FMS individual is the only one in the room who isn't wearing "real clothes." Everyone else may be wearing street clothes or even uniforms while he/she wears a gown. The other people are active, and at times being a "patient" requires being passive. The care givers give instructions, medicines, and therapy to the "patient." All of the above might imply that the patient does nothing important and that is inaccurate and demoralizing. Being a "patient" is only one of numerous roles and not an entire identity. Remember that when the doctor goes to the dentist he or she has that role. In the clinical setting, the FMS individual's job is to participate and become an active member of the team. When the "patient" clothing is shed, the individual's job is to go about the business of leading as full a life as possible. Being an active, involved and key member of the treatment plan is emotionally rewarding.

While doing so, it is important to keep in mind one critical distinction. Being a responsible "patient" and participating actively in self care does not mean that the FMS individual is to blame for having the illness in the first place. An FMS individual would never think such a cruel thing about someone with cancer or arthritis, so a reminder of "I didn't cause this" is important.

Anger

Anger is a common emotion when dealing with fibromyalgia. Feeling angry for a long time without discovering a way to safely express it or even acknowledge it is a burden. It is easier to talk about anger if there is a villain to target. When illness happens, anger is directed in many directions because usually there is no one responsible to direct it at. Many people have the idea that feeling angry is a bad thing. An individual can't help feeling an emotion, and experiencing it isn't the problem. The big problem is what is done with the feeling. Taking anger out on others is a harmful way to let the feelings out. Others are not responsible for what has occurred in the FMS individual's life.

Friendship

Companionship and friendship of friends and family is needed, and widespread resentment makes it difficult for these people to be close. Sometimes the worst outbursts of frustration and anger are inflicted on those who care for an FMS individual the most and are closest to him/her. They are the safest and most likely to still show love after the outburst. They are easily available targets for frustrated feelings and anger.

A sense of unfairness and fear of being dependent are often part of that anger. The fear of increased dependence causing those closest to an FMS individual to pull away is really frightening. Sadly, this fear can lead to behavior that makes it much more likely that the worst fears will be realized.

Acknowledge Facts

Anger turned inward is also not the answer. Anger turned inward often results in depression. Why is it so hard to handle this emotion with a chronic illness? Perhaps an individual confuses acceptance of the situation with liking what has happened. The angry feeling may be a way to let him/herself and the rest of the world know that this is really awful and it should go away. Accepting facts doesn't mean liking them or choosing the situation. Acceptance means working with reality and choosing to have more of life rather than less.

This brings back the subject of control. Genuine control is working with what an FMS individual has and not falling prey to the superman or victim role. Control helps perspective. Not only the person with fibromyalgia has bad and good days, so does everyone else. Before a person gets a diagnosis he/she can accept ups and downs in life as a matter of course, why not after? Having a bad spell is not justification for writing off the future. Plan for the future based on what can be done, not on what was possible in the past or on what should be done, or on what others do. Do not confuse this information with some glib slogan (make lemonade out of lemons). This is an attempt to overcome the real danger of giving up and settling for less than is deserved.

Anger as Motivation

Finding ways to use anger to motivate rather than block action, ways to appropriately ask for help and to say "no thank you" to offers of help, and ways to exercise control in life are some of the things to be learned. There are times when things aren't going well and the FMS individual feels sad and angry but be aware that those who care the most may feel inadequate or overwhelmed by the situation. An objective person who understands feelings but is not personally involved in the FMS individual's life is a safer person to talk with and is someone who can make observations that loved ones don't see or are afraid to mention.

Pets

If you do not have a pet, think seriously about getting one. Studies have shown that companion animals are beneficial to the physical and mental health of human beings. Walking a dog is the one form of exercise some individuals can do. It doesn't require club membership or a schedule with a friend to do it. There are less energetic interactions such as rolling a ball or dangling a ribbon for a cat. Always there is the company and affection of a living being happy for our companionship whether we are in a bad or good mood. If pets aren't allowed in your home or apartment, ask friends to share their animals or visit the humane society.

Spirituality

Spirituality is an important aspect in managing FMS. Spirituality is not defined as religion or going to church. Spirituality, or spiritual grounding, involves the concept of a higher supportive power. For some this is named God, for others Jehovah, for others Allah. Spirituality brings perspective to imperfection and suffering. It can help FMS individuals see the gifts of suffering, the gifts of limitations, and the progress of small slow steps forward and backward. Life for anyone is not a permanent uphill battle or celebration. Being in touch with your own spirit is a difficult course under any circumstances but especially when one is hurting. Finding quiet time for oneself, journaling, music, creative expression, connecting with close friends and family, sharing intimate thoughts and intimate moments – all these activities bring us closer to our spiritual self. This helps each individual with FMS find his/her own path through the depth of this illness. Spiritual grounding provides the base for the up and down path of FMS with a safety net under the "downs."

Guidelines

Judy, who has had fibromyalgia for six years, describes her priorities for staying emotionally healthy stating:

- Learn to say 'No' to things you don't want to do.
- Value your time and give some to yourself each day.
- Take time to exercise daily 20-30 minutes.
- Walk away from stressful situations that are not yours.
- Practice Physiological Quieting and meditation daily.

Chapter 22

What Can I Do
To Be Active At Home?

Joyce Dougan, P.T.
Janet A. Hulme, P. T.

The important tasks necessary for the function of a daily household can be overwhelming to someone who is in pain and feels fatigue. Household jobs are repetitive by nature so having a plan or schedule that prioritizes the FMS individual's comfort as equal importance to the day's endeavors is essential. Initially, list the week's jobs and distribute them over the seven days. Next, decide who will do each job, delegating to family members and hired help some of the tasks that cause the most pain and fatigue. Now, break up each task into smaller units and spread out the units through that day. For example, take rests between each room when vacuuming. Additionally, another job's sub task (chopping vegetables for dinner) can be done after the rest period and before the vacuuming is done again. Varying the tasks varies the muscles used and the movement patterns performed by the same muscles which decreases the possibility of pain and fatigue.

Cleaning

Spring house cleaning tasks should be hired out or spread throughout the year and involve the whole family. Yard work and gardening need to be low maintenance. Care free landscaping with evergreens, rocks and chips can be colorful with little care. Plastic under flower and vegetable gardens minimizes weeding. Use of raised beds saves strain on knees and back muscles. Pots of flowers or even vegetables can be placed in or out of the house and need minimal care.

Cooking

In the kitchen, organization of space and design can assist in comfortable meal preparation. Place frequently used objects within easy reach so there is minimal reaching overhead or a need to stoop to lift something. Pots and pans which are the heaviest need to be at the same level as the stove. Use a step stool to reach the cupboards that are overhead and sit on it to reach into the lowest cupboards. Whenever possible use light weight pots, pans, and dishes. Do food preparation seated at a table using an office chair with wheels rather than standing at the sink or counter. In the sink, raise the washing surface by placing a dish pan on top of four cups or plastic containers. At the counter use a thick cutting board or place equipment on 2x4s to elevate the work surface so there is minimal bending forward when working.

Planning meals a week at a time lets others help with grocery shopping on their days off. Carrying heavy bags to and from the car is a task where help is often needed. Have perishables bagged separately to take into the house immediately. Then get the rest later or let someone else help. Cooking meals using crock pots or making large portions of casseroles, lasagne or spaghetti can provide two days' meals instead of one. Planning one takeout meal or a frozen meal once a week gives the flexibility to not cook when a day has been particularly stressful. Buying children's cookbooks encourages them to cook a meal.

Laundry

Laundry is a task that can be aggravating to fibromyalgia symptoms unless pacing and simplification strategies are used. Wash one load a day instead of three or four a day. Let each family member do his/her own laundry when each is old enough to use the washing machine (9-10 years old). At least have family members sort their dirty clothes before someone washes and dries them, then they can pick up the clean clothes, fold and return them to their closets. Hire out ironing and buy wash and wear clothes. Underwear and sheets don't need ironing. Just fold underwear and lay sheets on the bed after drying. Have a basket of towels and washcloths unfolded that family members can use as they are needed. Those clothes that need folding can be folded on a counter top or while sitting at a table.

Bathroom

Bathroom cleaning can be simplified too. Clean and wipe down the tub after the shower or bath but while still in it. Use a long handled scrubber for reaching in the shower or tub to clean them. Wipe off the sink and toilet every other day as they are used. Use mild cleaning agents since some individuals are hypersensitive to chemicals.

Bill Paying

Bill paying and letter writing are more comfortable using a fine felt tipped pen on a slanted writing surface. When a computer keyboard is used, rest it on a pillow or lap board at elbow height in the lap. If the telephone is used much, a headset or speaker phone rather than manually holding the phone or securing the phone between the head and shoulder helps keep the FMS individual's neck and jaw from hurting.

Shopping

Shopping can be an exhausting event or a pleasurable experience depending on the planning that precedes the event. If walking and driving are problems, use mail order to purchase clothes, kitchen equipment, gifts, even shoes. Check on delivery services available in your area. Often they will do your shopping for you if you provide the list. Comparison shop by phone to find the best buys before making up a list. When planning to go out to shop, plan short trips and organize a list of items for different locations. Then go to one or two locations a day. Get a handicapped parking sticker from the local city/county offices. Use the wheelchairs or electric scooters available in stores. Say "yes" to offers of help in carrying shopping bags to the car. Ask if help isn't offered.

Travel

Traveling creates new challenges for the individual with FMS. The physical act of driving can take the pleasure out of traveling for someone with FMS. Taxis, buses, trains and planes can be used for travel without having to do the physical act of driving. Baggage assistance is usually available and should be utilized. Check all luggage and arrange door to door shuttle service to the destination before leaving home. Two small bags are better than one. Use a wheeled luggage cart to pull bags rather than carry them. When driving or riding in a car, well fitting back and arm supports are important. Get out, stretch and walk around frequently, usually at least every hour. For long trips, break up each day with longer rest periods by reclining in the back seat, visiting tourist sites while taking short walks, or having a picnic. Complete driving early in the day and stay where there is a hot tub and/or pool to use. When flying, use a small pillow for your low back. Use a blanket or sweater to keep drafts away from neck and shoulders. When staying over night away from home, have the pillow and eggcrate mattress from home. Remember to take sleep aids like ear plugs or a white noise machine. After arrival at the destination, pace the planned activities. Staying in one place and taking short side trips often works well. Keeping regular dietary habits and a medication schedule are important for an enjoyable vacation.

Chapter 23

What Can I Do To Successfully Work?

Joyce Dougan, P.T.
Ellen S. Silverglat, M.S.W.
Janet A. Hulme, P.T.

No examination of living with fibromyalgia is complete without looking at work. It is important to change the work environment because little things at work can result in enormous suffering later on. People working 40 hours per week spend approximately one third of the day on the job. It is likely that no other activity, including being with family and recreation, takes up such large blocks of time. Only the number of hours slept may approach the amount one works. Work is not only a big factor because of the amount of time spent at professions and employment, it is significant because of the reasons an individual works. In addition to providing financially for themselves and their dependents, an individual acquires part of their sense of identity from his/her work. In the best circumstances an FMS individual derives a sense of satisfaction from work that goes beyond the monetary compensation. The workplace is also an opportunity for socializing. Being able to continue to do one's work competently is of great concern to anyone with a chronic illness.

Pacing and Production

When an individual is concerned about being able to handle all of his/her duties there is often the urge to take a marathon approach to the job. This might include skipping breaks or lunch hours in order to spend as much time as possible "being productive." The same rationale may encourage overtime, not occasionally but routinely. This approach does not accomplish the desired goal, but it does affect the individual negatively. Quantity and quality of work actually decreases and the worker becomes less efficient. Typically it is common for the over-working individual to become more irritable, more fatigued and restless, and less positive about the work or his/her abilities. Anxiety about job performance can actually exacerbate the very symptoms one worries about interfering with performance.

There are approaches to doing one's job that can diminish fears and lessen tension. Take breaks on schedule. Use half of the fifteen minute break to loosen muscles, get fresh air, or chat about something not work related. At lunch time instead of eating at the desk or in the room, eat outside and take a walk after eating. Even running errands is probably better than feeling chained to the desk. If there isn't anyone to talk with, bring a book and read a chapter. Try using visualization techniques between tasks or on breaks. Use exercises the therapist outlined for breathing and relaxing specific muscles.

Interpersonal Relationships

Interpersonal relationships are a benefit of working but they can also be a stressor. Not all coworkers, peers and supervisors get along well. Personal problems, personality traits, and illness can affect how one relates to others. Spending a number of hours around someone difficult can be uncomfortable, but keeping the situation in perspective can help. Keep in mind that this person's primary role in your life is that of fellow employee, not friend. If working with a particular person is too stressful, talk to the personnel office or to the appropriate supervisor. It may be that at times the FMS individual blames illness for bad days when other factors that are hard to confront are a big part of the cause. Don't assume negative feelings are due to illness or medication. Having fibromyalgia or any other disease does not make someone exempt from everyday stressors.

Flareups and Work

What about those days when fibromyalgia flares up? Sometimes it is necessary to take sick days or time off for appointments. Even if the employer doesn't care about individual employee's health problems, it is usually a wise move to briefly explain the facts of the necessary treatment. Brief knowledge of the FMS individual's situation may make time for medical appointments less of an issue for co-workers and supervisors. Unless working with a good friend who will keep confidences, it is advisable not to discuss discomforts in great detail. Extensive descriptions of medical problems can get in the way of being viewed and treated as a peer. Remember everyone comes to the work place with some unique situation and hearing a lot about any one problem gets old.

Transition from Work to Home

Coming home from work is a time of transition, an adjustment from work to home. It is a good idea to allow a 30-60 minute period of time to make that transition. Some people read the mail, watch the news, change clothes, take a walk, or even grab a quick catnap. Ask family members to postpone non emergencies for the first 20 minutes to half hour so there is time to switch gears. This is a chance to let go of physical and mental stress from work and approach the role at home without that burden. If rest or a nap is needed after work, make a schedule that allows that routinely. The same rule applies to exercise or any other health maintenance routine. To help get the most out of the "quiet time" during the transition from work to home, have the evening meal prepared ahead of time. Solutions can be a crock pot or oven meal, a quick microwave meal or a takeout meal.

Adaptations

In the workplace there are many modifications to equipment, dress, and movement patterns that make the job easier and more efficient. Change positions frequently. For some individuals with FMS it will be necessary to change as often as every 15 minutes while for others every 30 minutes will be adequate. After sitting for a period of time, stand up and stretch or walk a short distance. After a time of standing, sit or walk for a short period. This change uses different muscle groups and decreases fatigue and pain.

For a standing job it is important to wear good supportive shoes. A building is only as good as its foundation and feet are the body's foundation. The work surface height is important in a standing job to protect the back. A general guideline is to have the surface approximately elbow height. Lifts can be put under table legs or legs can be cut off. A very simple and cost effective piece of equipment to increase standing tolerance is a rubberized floor mat. They are available through catalogues or in hardware, beauty supply houses, or restaurant supply stores.

If the primary work position is sitting, it is important to have a well fitted chair that offers good support for back and hips. The chair should allow the feet to be flat on the floor, the seat should be of adequate width to support the buttocks and thighs and deep enough so the seat ends about three inches from the back of the knee. The chair back should provide low back support to keep weight directly over ischial tuberosities or "butt bones." The shoulders and head will then more easily balance over the hips with less muscular effort. A high back chair with head and neck support is a choice for some individuals.

If work is performed while seated at a desk, the height of the desk and the position of the equipment on it are important considerations. The desk top should generally be at elbow height when sitting with back supported. If the desk is too high and requires shoulders and arms to be elevated all day there will be increased discomfort and decreased productivity.

If it isn't feasible to lower a desk the chair can be adjusted to a higher level with a foot rest added to keep the feet supported. When working on a computer the keyboard can often be put on a pullout shelf below the desktop to obtain the correct height.

Equipment location on a desk is important for the individual with FMS. Equipment used most often should be closest to the individual. This might mean rearranging the phone, calculator, rolodex, or computer. If the calculator is used frequently during the day, move it to midline so the individual's elbow can be at his/her side or resting on the desk when using the keyboard. Always have the computer monitor in midline at eye level 24 inches or one full arm's length away from your face. Eliminate glare on the screen. Position the keyboard close to the body and at approximately elbow height.

Some new equipment can decrease mechanical stresses on the job. A headset is essential if there is much phone work. Arm and wrist supports can be essential to improved production with less pain. A document holder can keep the head and neck comfortable when transposing data from documents to the computer.

Work Stress

The physical work environment - temperature, noise, lighting, and vibration – affects how the FMS individual feels and his/her productivity. These stressors can increase pain, stiffness and fatigue. If temperature is a problem, experiment with layering clothing and wearing silk turtlenecks, even in summer. If an air conditioning vent is positioned directly over the work area, check to see if it can be closed or angled differently or have a deflector placed on the vent. If noise is excessive, try ear plugs or use a headset with quiet music or nature sounds. Lighting can be angled differently or additional lighting can be added. Full spectrum overhead lights are more expensive but the cost is offset by the improved health and productivity of the employees. Rubber mats to stand on can absorb vibration. They can be put under desk and chair legs to decrease vibration from the environment to work surfaces.

In addition to having a good physical work setting, there is also the need to use the body efficiently. Learn to use only the muscles required for a task and keep the others relaxed. Use the necessary muscles as if they are floating through the task. Biofeedback can help achieve efficient muscle use first in the clinic and then at the job site. An ergonomic home specialist can help design the worksite.

Body Mechanics

Using good body mechanics during lifting, carrying, reaching, pushing and pulling is essential for comfort and efficiency. When lifting, it is recommended that feet be at least shoulder width apart and one slightly ahead of the other to provide a firm base of support. Bend knees, not the back, to get close to the item and lift while keeping the object close to the body. Keep the head up and exhale while lifting to help stabilize the back. When moving an item from one level to another (a laundry basket from floor to table) turn by walking rather than pivoting and twisting at the waist. Carrying with two hands is most effectively done with the weight held at waist level. When carrying an item at chest height the hips tend to lean forward to help maintain the individual's balance. This increases back strain. When carrying something in one hand at the side, like a 12 pack of pop, try to put something of comparable weight in the other hand for equal balance. When pushing an item, place one foot in front of the other so there is weight shift from the back foot to the front foot to initiate movement. Have the item to be pushed as directly in front of the body as possible to avoid twisting.

Job Changes and the ADA

At times it is necessary to change jobs, decrease the hours you work or not work at all for a period of time because of fibromyalgia symptoms. The physician, physical or occupational therapist, or vocational rehabilitation specialist can assist in analyzing the situation. Part time work may be an option, a change in job description, or a new job that better fits the individual's needs are options to consider. Sometimes self employment is the best choice for the FMS individual since he/she can work at his/her own pace and accept contracts that are doable. Retraining, education for a new occupation, and career counseling are all options to consider when the present job is not the best alternative.

The Americans with Disability Act (ADA) describes that a qualified individual with a disability who can perform the essential functions of his/her job cannot be discriminated against. The employer is required to make reasonable accommodations for the worker unless it would impose undue hardship.

Chapter 24

What Can I Do To Have Fun And Play?

Joyce Dougan, P.T.
Ellen S. Silverglat, M.S.W.
Janet A. Hulme, P.T.

Fun and play are part of every individual's balanced lifestyle. The individual with fibromyalgia has the need for fun and play as much or more than anyone else. Many times when asked "What do you do for fun?" the FMS individual responds "I work" or "I don't have time for fun and play." The idea that work is what is really important and play is a sideline for the lazy can be replaced with the idea that there needs to be a balance of work, play, and rest to be healthy. Some FMS individuals describe waiting to play until the pain is gone or until a new medicine is found to cure them before they play. Instead the FMS individual must look for the new medicine but continue to have balance in everyday life through fun and play. The thought that play and leisure is a luxury of the past and no longer a possibility with FMS can be replaced with the idea that play and leisure are a necessity, not a luxury. Sometimes FMS individuals respond "I might injure myself or make things worse; I'm too fragile now." The replacement thought is "I can learn to play safely."

Fear of Failure

Sometimes the fear of failure gets in the way of fun and play. The FMS individual thinks, "I must be able to play the way I did before." The replacement thought is, "There is more than one way to enjoy myself and the search for the new ways can be fun." Some FMS individuals say, "Competition is the key, without it there is no point in a recreational activity. Those other activities are for wimps." The replacement thought pattern can be, "Really? Wouldn't something be better than nothing?" The thought that "I can't learn a new activity now that I have this problem" sometimes puts a roadblock up to fun and play. The question to ask is "Have I tried? What do I have to lose?"

What is Possible

The individual with FMS must focus on what he/she can realistically do. Instead of the thought, "I can't run 5 miles a day so I won't do anything" say, "I can go for walks with friends along the river." Instead of the thought, "I'll swim 3000 yards even if I can't get out of bed tomorrow," say, "I'll do water aerobics for 30 minutes in a warm pool." The focus is on what the individual can do in comfort and without extreme fatigue while having fun and "playing."

Redefining Fun and Play

Redefining fun and play is a gradual process. The exercise to "Think of what you did as a child, then as an adolescent for fun and play. What activities that you did then might be fun now?" is often helpful in coming up with 'new ideas' for fun and play. As a child you painted pictures and admired them. By suspending judgment and just "doing," the joy of noncompetitive fun returns.

Another question to ask is, "What are the fun and play activities I've always thought I might try? How can I modify them so I can enjoy the new event and feel OK the next day?" There is never a better time to find out how to do something new. Maybe it's archery or horseback riding that interests you. Plan to take lessons from a professional and adjust the time spent to your energy and pain level. If the roadblock is "I might get too tired or sore and have to go slow or even stop for awhile" discuss this with the instructor and plan rest periods ahead of time. Developing new hobbies can add variety to leisure time. New crafts, bird watching, flower arranging, photography, collecting old toy trucks at garage sales, are all possibilities. Using a computer to make new friends and to play computer games can be a whole new world. Dream about what might be interesting and fun. Then try it!

Pacing Play

Often the question of, "How do I go on excursions with friends when I know I won't be able to keep up with them?" comes up. The solution may be to plan parallel play with meeting places along the way for conversation and meals. For example, on a cross-country ski excursion with friends, the FMS individual may go at his/her pace with frequent rests while the others are on a more difficult trail at a faster pace but there is a planned meeting time and place for lunch to compare notes and enjoy the company. When vacations are planned, the FMS individual may plan to fly to the destination while others drive.

Plan Ahead

In all leisure and play, plan ahead to make the event pleasant. Get a doctor's prescription and obtain a handicapped parking permit and find out where the parking area is. Take a back cushion or special chair when the event requires sitting. Sit at the end of the aisle so you can get up and move around. Use a stadium seat if the event's seating is on bleachers. Take a change of clothes or wear layers for the possibility of weather and temperature changes. Take healthy snacks and water.

Entertaining at home means preparing food several days ahead of time or having meals catered. Housecleaning can also be done ahead and delegated to family members or hired out. The day before the event it is important to plan rest periods interspersed in the day's work. During the event having a quiet place to spend five minutes resting can help make the event pleasant for you as well as the guests.

A Positive Outlook

Creating a positive outlook about leisure activities means building a thought framework to support fun. Expecting to enjoy yourself whether alone or in the company of others is a part of fun and leisure. Changing negative thoughts to positive "I can try" thoughts is essential. Avoiding tunnel vision about what is a fun activity and enjoying many aspects of any activity lets fun come into everyday life. Everyone benefits from enjoying the process, the path, not just the end result of leisure and fun activities.

Rest beforehand, rest along the way, learn pacing with the idea of not hurting the next day. Discuss with companions and family the "comfort zone" of activity. Build up gradually in endurance over a two to three month period. Know that fun and play are their own reward. Fun and play are as important to schedule as work and rest.

Chapter 25

What Can My Family Do To Help?

Ellen S. Silverglat, M.S.W.
Janet A. Hulme, P.T.

Families become involved in the FMS individual's care, attitude, and goals. Family members need to become educated about fibromyalgia. It isn't simple to explain, but it is worth the effort. Explain to family members that, "yes, it is real, no there is no cure for it, and yes I can deal with it. I wish it would go away too, but it won't."

Let family members know there will be bad days and good days. "I will be as active as is possible and as is good for me." A mother will explain, "some days you may have to iron your own shirt or make your own lunch."

Understand that a "bad mood" may be a part of fibromyalgia or it may just be a bad mood. This illness doesn't explain everything about the individual. "The same stuff that irritated me before bothers me now. The same things that delighted me before please me now."

Relax, a person with fibromyalgia won't break. "I am not an invalid. I am not dying. Some days I am more incapacitated than others, some days I need more attention than others. You can help by doing more for yourself but I am still your wife, mother, daughter, or son."

Fibromyalgia is an illness, not an excuse. "None of us should use it to explain away things. All of us need to be honest."

The symptoms of fibromyalgia are real – headaches, back pain, gut pain, fatigue, confusion – all are real, they come and go. "Please don't pretend my symptoms don't exist, don't ridicule me or put me down when I tell you how I feel. Just say I hear you, it's not your fault."

Families learn that doing less may mean being able to do more in the case of someone with fibromyalgia. Daily schedules let the family know what activity limits there are and when there are rest times scheduled. Then there is not the need for a family member to ask "Are you sure you want to do this?" or "Do you feel so bad you need to take a break?"

Family members need reassurance that you are in control. "I don't need a keeper. I'm happy being quiet sometimes. I'm responsible for seeing to my own health care. I'll ask for help when I need it."

Half a loaf is better than none in the case of fibromyalgia. "I can feel sorry for myself if I need to, but don't encourage it. I'll take advantage of opportunities to live my life to the fullest. Thank you for your support."

Care but please don't hover or try to disprove how the individual with FMS feels or believes. "If I need to hibernate, don't rebut me. If you read an article in a magazine that says fibromyalgia is due to poor spiritual life, don't be eager to tell me. If your best friend's aunt who has fibromyalgia dropped dead . . . or ate a diet of dandelions and never ached again . . . or joined a cult to deal with fibromyalgia, please understand that I may be disinclined to do the same." Illnesses of unknown cause invite unproved remedies. Don't undermine the treatments that are trusted and comfortable for the individual with fibromyalgia.

"When I whine, just say you are sorry it's a bad day and you hope things will improve. They will."

"Let me care for you when you aren't feeling well. It's important to be able to give back."

Coaching and a Circle of Support

Everyone needs a circle of support to accomplish their life goals. When fibromyalgia is a consideration in daily life it is important that the circle of support is focused on:

- where the individual with FMS wants to go
- what the individual with FMS dreams of being
- quality of life goals

- incremental steps to move toward the goals
- positive motivation

Quality of life goals are very different than accomplishment/measurement goals. Quality of life goals look at improvement in:

- daily life skills
- social and recreational possibilities
- mental frame of reference skills

Accomplishment/measurement goals direct an individual with FMS to compare performance today with yesterday and with others' behavior. Since FMS is a chronic condition and there are variations in symptom severity, measurement related goals are not conducive to long term improvement.

The circle of support can include family members, friends, medical personnel, internet friends, relatives, and work acquaintences. Their responsibility is to understand FMS and your goals. Their role is to approach your support through a wellness model. The message is continually "This is where you are. This is where you want to go. You have the ability to take care of yourself and move toward those goals. Sometimes the going will be slow, sometimes faster, but always there is the motivation to keep your eye on the prize." Hope, dreams, and small baby steps are what a circle of support is made of.

Listening is a function of the circle of support. Listening to what is good, what is being attempted, what has been accomplished, what problems the individual is encountering. When negativity creeps into the conversation the response is, "That's really terrible. What can you do about it?" A circle of support is a positive coaching group with realistic ideas and an empowering attitude.

Encouragement is a function of the circle of support. The individual with FMS says "I'm tired of this self care, what good does it do anyway?" The response is, "Are you still having severe headaches, sleeplessness, (previous symptoms)? The self care you have done has improved your life." When a person complains he/she is really asking for helpful encouragement.

Notes:

Chapter 25: What Can My Family Do To Help?

My Master Test and
Self Care Stabilizing Protocol

Tests: Date																	
1.																	
2.																	
3.																	
4.																	
Self Care Protocol																	
1.																	
2.																	
3.																	
4.																	
5.																	
6.																	
7.																	
8.																	
9.																	
10.																	

Notes:

References

Chapter One

Donaldson CC et al: Disinhibition in the gamma motorneuron circuitry: a neglected mechanism for understanding myofascial pain syndromes? Applied Psychophysiology & Biofeedback 23#1:43-57, 1998.

Chapter Two

Jacobsen S et al: Musculoskeletal Pain, Myofascial Pain Syndrome, and the Fibromyalgia Syndrome. New York: Haworth Medical Press, 1993.

Chapter Three

Childre D et al: The Heartmath Solution. San Francisco: HarperCollins, 1999.

Cutler W, Garcia C: Menopause A Guide for Women and the Men Who Love Them (revised). New York: WW Norton & Co, 1992.

Fried R: The Hyperventilation Syndrome: Research and Clinical Treatment. Baltimore: John Hopkins University Press, 1987.

Gershon M: The Second Brain, New York: HarperCollins, 1998.

Goldstein J et al: Betrayal of the Brain: The Neurologic Basis of Chronic Fatigue Syndrome, Fibromyalgia Syndrome and Related Neural Network Disorders. Binghampton, NY: Haworth Press, 1996.

Griep EN et al: Altered reactivity of the HPA axis in the primary fibromyalgia syndrome. Jrnl of Rheum 20:469-474, 1993.

Hendricks G: Conscious Breathing. New York: Bantam Books, 1995.

Ornish D: Love and Survival The Scientific Basis for the Healing Power of Intimacy. New York: HarperCollins, 1997.

Pellegrino MJ et al: Familial occurrence of primary fibromyalgia. Arch Phys Med Rehabil 70:61-63, 1989.

Pert C: Molecules of Emotion. The Science Behind Mind-Body Medicine. New York: Simon & Schuster, 1997.

Slagle P: The Way Up From Down. New York: Random House, 1987.

Teitelbaum J: From Fatigued to Fantastic A Manual for Moving Beyond Chronic Fatigue and Fibromyalgia. Garden City Park, NY: Avery Publishing, 1996.

Yunus, MB et al: A study of multicase families with fibromyalgia with HLA typing. Arthritis Rheum 35:S285, 1992.

Chapter Four

Hulme J, Penner B: Chronic Pain: Assessment and Lifetime Strategies for Fibromyalgia. Eighth Annual Congress on Women's Health and Gender Based Medicine. Hilton Head, SC June 3-6, 2000.

Jacobsen S et al: Musculoskeletal Pain, Myofascial Pain Syndrome, and the Fibromyalgia Syndrome. New York: Haworth Medical Press, 1993.

Chapter Eight

Tyler V: Honest Herbal. New York: Haworth Press, 1993.

Yao J: Acutherapy Acupuncture T.E.N.S. and Acupressure. Libertyville, IL: Acutherapy Postgraduate Seminars, 1984.

Chapter Nine

Turaccioli G et al: EMG-biofeedback training in fibromyalgia syndrome. J Rheum 14: 820-825, 1987.

Chapter Eleven

Genter P, Ipp E: Plasma glucose thresholds for counterregulation after an oral glucose load. Metabolism 43 #1 (Jan 1994) 98-103.

Wilson E: Wilson's Syndrome. Orlando Fl: Cornerstone Publishing. 1996.

Chapter Twelve

Bremer HJ et al: Disturbances of Amino Acid Metabolism. Baltimore: Urban & Schwarzenberg, 1981.

Bueler P: Talking to Yourself. San Francisco: HarperCollins, 1991.

Lieberman S, Bruning N: The Real Vitamin & Mineral Book. Garden City Park, NY: Avery Publishing, 1997.

Ornstein R, Sobel D: Healthy Pleasures. New York: Addison-Wesley Publishing, 1989.

Penner B: Managing Fibromyalgia. A Six-Week Course on Self Care. Missoula, MT: Phoenix Publishing, 1997.

Pert C: Molecules of Emotion. The Science Behind Mind-body Medicine. New York: Simon & Schuster, 1997.

Slagle P: The Way Up From Down. New York: Random House, 1987.

Travell J, Simons D: Myofascial Pain & Dsyfunction The Trigger Point Mnaual. Baltimore: Williams & Wilkins, 1983.

Yao J: Acutherapy Acupuncture T.E.N.S. and Acupressure. Libertyville, IL: Acutherapy Postgraduate Seminars, 1984.

Chapter Fourteen

Cathey MA, et al: Functional ability and work status in patients with fibromyalgia. Arthritis Care and Research 1:2: 85-98, 1988.

Hulme J, Penner B: Chronic Pain: Assessment and Lifetime Strategies for Fibromyalgia. Eighth Annual Congress on Women's Health and Gender Based Medicine. Hilton Head, SC, June 3-6, 2000.

Jacobsen S et al: Musculoskeletal Pain, Myofascial Pain Syndrome, and the Fibromyalgia Syndrome. New York: Haworth Medical Press, 1993.

Silverman S, Mason J: Measuring the functional impact of fibromyalgia. J Musculoskel Med 9:7: 15-24, 1992.

Chapter Fifteen

Amand P, Marek C: What Your Doctor May Not Tell You About Fibromyalgia. New York: Warner Books, 1999.

Genter P, Ipp E: Plasma glucose thresholds for counterregulation after an oral glucose load. Metabolism 43 #1: 98-103, Jan 1994.

Sears B: Enter the Zone. New York: HarperCollins Publishing, 1995.

Chapter Sixteen

Balch F, Balch P: Prescription for Nutritional Healing, 2nd ed. Garden City, NY: Avery Publishing, 1997.

Barnes BO: Hypothyroidism, The Unsuspected Illness. New York: Harper & Row, 1976.

Pearsall P: The Heart's Code. New York: Broadway Books, 1998.

Slagle P: The Way Up From Down. New York: Random House, 1987.

Wilson E: Wilson's Syndrome. Orlando Fl: Cornerstone Publishing. 1996

Chapter Seventeen

Rowe PC et al: Is neurally mediated hypotension an unrecognized cause of chronic fatigue syndrome. Lancet 345: 623-624, march 11, 1995.

Teitelbaum J: From Fatigued to Fantastic A Manual for Moving Beyond Chronic Fatigue and Fibromyalgia. Garden City Park, NY: Avery Publishing, 1996.

Chapter Eighteen

Crook W: Chronic Fatigue and the Yeast Connection. Jackson, TN: Professional Books, 1992.

Peter JB: Abnormal immune regulation in fibromyalgia. Arthritis Rheum 31:524, 1988.

Stermberg EM: Hypoimmune fatigue syndromes: disease of the stress response Jrnl of Rheum 20: 418-421 editorial (1993).

Chapter Nineteen

Abraham GE: Nutrition and the premenstrual tension syndromes. Jrnl of Applied Nutrition 36:2:103-17, 1984.

Bzulieu E et al. DHEA, DHEA sulfate and aging: contribution of the DHEA Age study to a sociobiomedical issue. Proc Natl. Acad. Sci. 97 #8: 4279-4284, April 2000.

Crapo L: Hormones The Messengers of Life, Stanford, Ca: Stanford Alumni Assoc, 1985.

Cutler W, Garcia C: Menopause A Guide for Women and the Men Who Love Them (revised). New York: WW Norton & Co, 1992.

Diamond J: Male Menopause. Naperville, Il: Sourcebooks Inc, 1997.

Maizner W: Gender and Pain. University of North Carolina, Chapel Hill, NC: American Pain Society 1998.

Sahelian R: DHEA A Practical Guide. Garden City Park, NY: Avery Publishing, 1996.

Teitelbaum J: From Fatigued to Fantastic A Manual for Moving Beyond Chronic Fatigue and Fibromyalgia. Garden City Park, NY: Avery Publishing, 1996.

Yue SK: Relaxin: Its Role in the Pathogenesis of Fibromyalgia. http://www.relaxin.org/relaxinarticle. Dec 5-6, 1997.

Chapter Twenty

Hulme J, Penner B: Chronic Pain: Assessment and Lifetime Strategies for Fibromyalgia. Eighth Annual Congress on Women's Health and Gender Based Medicine. Hilton Head, SC, June 3-6, 2000.

Jacobsen S et al: Musculoskeletal Pain, Myofascial Pain Syndrome, and the Fibromyalgia Syndrome. New York: Haworth Medical Press, 1993.

Chapter Twenty One

Pitzele, S: We Are Not Alone Learning to Live With Chronic Illness. New York: Workman Publishing, 1986.

Product Sources

Personal Monitor Kit for Fibromyalgia

Blood Glucose Monitor
Basal Body Temperature Monitor and Hand Temperature Monitor
Blood Pressure and Heart Rate Monitor

Phoenix Inc.
(800) 549-8371
www.phoenixpub.com

Personal Care Kit for Fibromyalgia

Exercise Plan
Physiological Quieting Audiotape
Weekly Diary

Massage Oil
Self Care Book
Thermister

Phoenix Inc.
(800) 549-8371
www.phoenixpub.com

Nutritional Supplements

Melaleuca Vitamin Supplements
    Fructose based vitamin/mineral supplements
    (800) 549-8371
Nutritec
    Amino acid/vitamin/mineral supplements
    (800) 235-5727
Ideal Health
    Customized amino acid/vitamin/mineral supplements based on
    in-home metabolic testing
    (800) 549-8371

Biofeedback EMG Home Unit   Hot/Cold Therapy

Surface EMG rental unit
Phoenix, Inc.
(800) 549-8371

Cold Cups, Sticks, Wraps
Banner Therapy Products
(888) 277-1188

Stretching and Exercise Videos

Sit and Be Fit
P.O. Box 8033
Spokane, WA 99203

Fibromyalgia Fitness Videos
Oregon Fibromyalgia Foundation
1221 SW Yamhill, Ste. 303
Portland, OR 97205
www.myalgia.com

Chemically Sensitive Products

www.guiadoc.com
www.andrearose.com

Websites

Arthritis Foundation
http://www.arthritis.org/

American College of Rheumatology
http://www.rheumatology.org/

Association of Rheumatology Health
http://www.rheumatology.org/arhp/

The American Fibromyalgia Syndrome Association, Inc.
http://www.afsafund.org/

International Myopain Society
http://www.myopain.org/

National Institute for Arthritis and Musculoskeletal and Skin Diseases
http://www.nih.gov/niams/healthinfo/fibrofs.htm/

The American Pain Society
http://www.ampainsoc.org/

Drug Search from First Data Bank
http://www.medscape.com/misc/formdrugs.html

Organizations

Arthritis Foundation
1314 Spring Street, NW
Atlanta, Georgia 30309
(800) 283-7800

Fibromyalgia Alliance of America
P.O. Box 21990
Columbus, OH 43221
614-457-4222

Fibromyalgia Network
P.O. Box 31750
Tucson, AZ 85751
(800) 853-2929

National Chronic Fatigue and Fibromyalgia Syndrome Assoc.
P.O. Box 18426
Kansas City, MO 64133
816-931-4777

ORDER FORM

I would like to order additional copies of
Fibromyalgia, A Handbook for Self Care and Treatment

1-9 Copies $14.95 ea.   •   10 or more copies $10.95 ea.

No. of copies_____   x **$14.95** =   _____

No. of copies_____   x **$10.95** =   _____

Shipping & Handling (1st copy)   = $ **3.50**

Each additional copy **$1.00**   = $ _____

Total Cost of Order _____ $ _____

Please send check or money order to:

Phoenix Publishing Co.
P.O. Box 8231
Missoula, MT 59807
1-800-549-8371

www.phoenixpub.com

Name_____

Address _____

City_____State____Zip _____

Telephone (_____) _____